American Journal of Nephrology

Founded 1981 and edited until 2002 by S.G. Massry

KARGER

Printed in Switzerland
on acid-free paper by
Reinhardt Druck, Basel

Appears bimonthly:
1 volume per year
(6 issues)

Guidelines for Authors

American Journal of Nephrology

Submission

The 'American Journal of Nephrology' only accepts online submissions to:
www.rapidreview.com/AJN2/CALogon.jsp
All further technical instructions can be found there.

Conditions

The journal will not publish articles which have been previously reported at any length or articles being considered for publication elsewhere. The authors must include a statement to this effect in their cover letter. If publication of the data in any form has occurred or is being contemplated, a copy of such publication should be included with the submitted manuscript. Submission of an article for publication implies the transfer of the copyright from the author to the publisher upon acceptance. It is the author's responsibility to obtain permission to reproduce illustrations, tables, etc. from other publications. The manuscript should be written in English and the editors reserve the right to make appropriate corrections in grammar and style. Accepted papers become the permanent property of the 'American Journal of Nephrology' and may not be reproduced by any means, in whole or in part, without the written consent of the publisher. Information concerning financial disclosures (i.e. grants, funding, support, etc.) should be placed at the foot of the title page.

Types of Articles

Two types of articles will be accepted:
(a) Original Reports: Representing full sets of completed experiments that answer a given question. Max. 2,000 words, excl. figures, tables and references.
(b) In-Depth Topic Reviews: Covering a timely topic by experts in the field. Max. 4,000 words, excl. figures, tables and references.

The new focus of the journal is on basic science papers. The journal is no longer encouraging clinical papers such as case reports and small studies unless they pursue mechanisms of a disease process. All other manuscripts will be returned to the authors.

Page charges
Original Reports exceeding the first 5 printed pages which are free will cost USD 275.00 per extra page.

Arrangement

Title page: The first page of each paper should indicate the title, the authors' names, the institute where the work was conducted, and a short title for use as running head.
NB: Authors wishing to preserve the phonetic meaning of diacritics (PubMed reduces diacritics to their root characters) must spell their names accordingly when submitting manuscripts (e.g. Müller should be Mueller).

Full address: The exact postal address of the corresponding author complete with postal code must be given at the bottom of the title page. Please also supply phone and fax numbers, as well as e-mail address.

Key words: For indexing purposes, a list of 3–10 key words in English is essential.

Abstract: Each paper needs an abstract of up to 200 words. It should be structured as follows:

Background/Aims:	What is the major problem that prompted the study?
Methods:	How was the study performed?
Results:	Most important findings?
Conclusion:	Most important conclusion?

Footnotes: Avoid footnotes.

Tables and illustrations: Tables and illustrations (both numbered in Arabic numerals) should be prepared on separate pages. Tables require a heading and figures a legend, also prepared on a separate page. Electronically submitted b/w half-tone and color illustrations must have a final resolution of 300 dpi after scaling, line drawings one of 800–1,200 dpi.

Color Illustrations

The 'American Journal of Nephrology' gives you the choice to publish your color illustrations in the following manner:

Full color: Color illustrations are reproduced online and in print. Up to 6 color illustrations per page can be integrated within the text at the special price of CHF/USD 760.00 per page.

Online only: Color illustrations are reproduced free of charge online. In the print version, the illustrations are reproduced in black and white. Please avoid referring to the colors in the text and figure legends.

References

In the text identify references by Arabic numerals [in square brackets]. Material submitted for publication but not yet accepted should be noted as 'unpublished data' and not be included in the reference list. The list of references should include only those publications which are cited in the text. Do not alphabetize; number references in the order in which they are first mentioned in the text. The surnames of the authors followed by initials should be given. There should be no punctuation other than a comma to separate the authors. Preferably, cite all authors. Abbreviate journal names according to the Index Medicus system. (Also see International Committee of Medical Journal Editors: Uniform requirements for manuscripts submitted to biomedical journals. N Engl J Med 1997;336:309–315. www.icmje.org)

Digital Object Identifier (DOI)
S. Karger Publishers supports DOIs as unique identifiers for articles. A DOI number will be printed on the title page of each article. DOIs can be useful in the future for identifying and citing articles published online without volume or issue information. More information can be found at www.doi.org.

Examples
(a) Papers published in periodicals: Chatel J-M, Bernard H, Orson FM: Isolation and characterization of two complete Ara h 2 isoforms cDNA. Int Arch Allergy Immunol 2003;131:14–18.
(b) Papers published only with DOI numbers:
Theoharides TC, Boucher W, Spear K: Serum interleukin-6 reflects disease severity and osteoporosis in mastocytosis patients. Int Arch Allergy Immunol DOI: 10.1159/000063858.
(c) Monographs: Matthews DE, Farewell VT: Using and Understanding Medical Statistics, ed 3, revised. Basel, Karger, 1996.
(d) Edited books: DuBois RN: Cyclooxygenase-2 and colorectal cancer; in Dannenberg AJ, Dubois RN (eds): COX-2. Prog Exp Tum Res. Basel, Karger, 2003, vol 37, pp 124–137.

Proofs

Unless indicated otherwise, proofs are sent to the corresponding author and should be returned with the least possible delay. Alterations made in proofs, other than the correction of printer's errors, are charged to the author.

Reprints

Order forms and a price list are sent with the proofs. Orders submitted after the issue is printed are subject to considerably higher prices.

KARGER

Fax +41 61 306 12 34
E-Mail karger@karger.ch
www.karger.com

The Guidelines for Authors are available at:
www.karger.com/ajn_Guidelines

General Information

American Journal of Nephrology

Publication data: 'American Journal of Nephrology' is published 6 times a year. Volume 25 with 6 issues appears in 2005.

Subscription rates: Subscriptions run for a full calendar year. Prices are given per year.

Personal subscription:

Print or Online	Print/Online combined
CHF 390.20	CHF 431.20
EUR 289.–	EUR 319.–
USD 317.20	USD 350.20
postage and handling	(added to print and print/online)
CHF 32.70 Europe,	CHF 48.60 Overseas
EUR 23.70	
USD 32.70	

Institutional subscription:

Print or Online	Print/Online combined
CHF 1951.–	CHF 2107.–
EUR 1445.–	EUR 1561.–
USD 1586.00	USD 1713.00
postage and handling	(added to print and print/online)
CHF 40.80 Europe,	CHF 60.60 Overseas
EUR 29.40	
USD 40.80	

Airmail surcharge: CHF 40.80 / USD 33.90

Microforms: Please direct all enquiries and orders to:
University Microfilms Inc.
300 North Zeeb Road, P.O. Box 1346
Ann Arbor, MI 48106-1346 (USA)

Subscription orders: Orders can be placed at agencies, bookstores, directly with the Publisher
S. Karger AG, P.O. Box
CH–4009 Basel (Switzerland)
or with any of the following distributors:
Deutschland: S. Karger GmbH, Postfach
D–79095 Freiburg
France: Librairie Luginbühl
36, bd de Latour-Maubourg
F–75007 Paris
Great Britain, Ireland: S. Karger AG
4 Rickett Street
London SW6 1RU, UK
USA: S. Karger Publishers, Inc.
26 West Avon Road, P.O. Box 529
Farmington, CT 06085, USA
India, Bangladesh, Sri Lanka:
Panther Publishers Private Ltd.
33, First Main
Koramangala First Block
Bangalore 560 034, India
Japan: Karger Japan, Inc.
Yushima S Bld. 3F
4-2-3, Yushima, Bunkyo-ku
Tokyo 113-0034, Japan

Change of address: Both old and new address should be sent to the subscription source.

Single issues and back volumes: Information can be obtained through the Publisher.

Advertising: Correspondence and rate requests should be addressed to the Publisher.

Bibliographic indices: This journal is regularly listed in bibliographic services, including *Current Contents®* and Index Medicus/MEDLINE.

Book Reviews: Books are accepted for review by special agreement.

Copying: This journal has been registered with the Copyright Clearance Center (CCC), as indicated by the code appearing on the first page of each article. For readers in the US, this code signals consent for copying of articles for personal or internal use, or for the personal or internal use of specific clients, provided that the stated fee is paid per copy directly to
Copyright Clearance Center Inc.
222 Rosewood Drive
Danvers, MA 01923 (USA)
A copy of the first page of the article must accompany payment. Consent does not extend to copying for general distribution, for promotion, for creating new works, or for resale. In these cases, specific written permission must be obtained from the copyright owner,
S. Karger AG,
P.O. Box, CH–4009 Basel (Switzerland).

KARGER

Fax +41 61 306 12 34
E-Mail karger@karger.ch
www.karger.com

The Journal Home Page is available at:
www.karger.com/ajn

American Journal of Nephrology

Am J Nephrol 2005;25(suppl 1):1–28
DOI: 10.1159/000082974

Published online: February 21, 2005

Dietary Management of Chronic Kidney Disease Patients: Protein-Restricted Diets Supplemented with Keto/Amino Acids

Abstracts
from the International Advisory Board Meetings 2003/2004

International Advisory Board
Michel Aparicio, Bordeaux, France
Rubén Darío Bonilla Aguirre, Guadalajara, Mexico
Adamasco Cupisti, Pisa, Italy
Sergio Draibe, São Paulo, Brazil
Shantan Lin, Shanghai, China
William E. Mitch, Atlanta, Ga., USA
Vladimír Teplan, Prague, Czech Republic
Gabor Zakar, Székesfehérvár, Hungary

Guest
Hans-Jürgen Schober-Halstenberg, Berlin, Germany

14 figures and 5 tables, 2005

KARGER

Basel · Freiburg · Paris · London · New York · Bangalore · Bangkok · Singapore · Tokyo · Sydney

S. Karger
Medical and Scientific Publishers
Basel • Freiburg • Paris • London
New York • Bangalore • Bangkok
Singapore • Tokyo • Sydney

Drug Dosage
The authors and the publisher have exerted every effort to ensure that drug selection and dosage set forth in this text are in accord with current recommendations and practice at the time of publication. However, in view of ongoing research, changes in government regulations, and the constant flow of information relating to drug therapy and drug reactions, the reader is urged to check the package insert for each drug for any change in indications and dosage and for added warnings and precautions. This is particularly important when the recommended agent is a new and/or infrequently employed drug.

P.O. Box, CH–4009 Basel (Switzerland)
Printed in Switzerland on acid-free paper by
Reinhardt Druck, Basel
ISBN 3–8055–7919–5

KARGER

Fax +41 61 306 12 34
E-Mail karger@karger.ch
www.karger.com

Vol. 25, Suppl. 1, 2005

American Journal of Nephrology

Contents

5 **Editorial**
Mitch, W.E. (Atlanta, Ga.)

Abstracts

Keto Acid Therapy in CKD Patients

6 **Epidemiology of CKD Worldwide**
Schober-Halstenberg, H.-J. (Berlin)

7 **Dietary Therapy in CKD Patients – The Current Status**
Mitch, W.E. (Atlanta, Ga.)

8 **Keto/Amino Acids in the Treatment of Chronic Kidney Disease Patients: 30 Years Experience in 3,000 Patients**
Teplan, V. (Prague)

10 **Eight Years of Ketosteril® Treatment in Hungary**
Zakar, G. (Székesfehérvàr)

10 **Overview of the Uremia Program**
Draibe, S. (São Paulo)

12 **The Pisa Experience on the Use of Keto Acids in Nephrology**
Cupisti, A. (Pisa)

13 **The Chronic Kidney Disease in Mexico**
Bonilla Aguirre, R.D. (Guadalajara)

13 **Pharmacological Features of a Keto Amino Acid Therapy**
Teplan, V. (Prague)

15 **Nephrology in China**
Lin, S. (Shanghai)

15 **Are Supplemented Low-Protein Diets Nutritionally Safe?**
Aparicio, M. (Bordeaux)

16 **Consensus: Keto Acid Therapy in CKD Patients**
International Advisory Board

Keto Acid Therapy for Patients with Diabetic Nephropathy

17 **Risk of Developing ESRD in Patients with Diabetic Nephropathy-Lessons from the USA**
Mitch, W.E. (Atlanta, Ga.)

18 **Standards of Care for Diabetic Nephropathy**
Teplan, V. (Prague)

21 **Place of Dietary Protein Restriction in the Treatment of Diabetic Nephropathy**
Aparicio, M. (Bordeaux)

23 **Italy – Clinical Studies on Protein Restriction in Diabetic Nephropathy Patients – Keto Acid Therapy and Its Efficacy**
Cupisti, A. (Pisa)

24 **Predialytic Treatment in CKD Patients**
Bonilla Aguirre, R.D. (Guadalajara)

25 **Consensus: Keto Acid Therapy for Patients with Diabetic Nephropathy**
International Advisory Board

Keto Acid Supplementation in Patients Being Treated by Dialysis

26 **Nutritional Requirement during Long-Term Dialysis Treatment and Nutritional Status of Dialysis Patients – What Is the Optimal Amount of Protein?**
Draibe, S. (São Paulo)

27 **Clinical Studies on Keto/Amino Acid Supplementation of Dialysis Patients**
Zakar, G. (Székesfehérvàr)

28 **Consensus: Keto Acid Supplementation in Patients Being Treated by Dialysis**
International Advisory Board

KARGER

Fax +41 61 306 12 34
E-Mail karger@karger.ch
www.karger.com

Access to full text and tables of contents, including tentative ones for forthcoming issues: www.karger.com/ajn_issues

Fresenius Kabi
Caring for Life

Publication of this issue was made possible by Fresenius Kabi.

Editorial

American Journal of Nephrology

Introduction and Goals of the International Advisory Board Meetings

Prediction at the end of the year 2002 suggest that the number of people undergoing dialysis will increase to a number far greater than predicted in earlier years. The prevalence of end-stage renal disease (ESRD) continues to grow throughout the world. This growth is driven by an aging population, an increased incidence of diseases associated with kidney damage (especially diabetes), and greater access to dialysis therapy. The costs of treating ESRD patients also is growing and represents a difficult economic problem throughout the world and this could lead to economic factors that impose restrictions on treatment. In short, new methods of preventing and treating chronic kidney disease (CKD) are required.

It has been known for over 130 years that dietary protein restriction is a critical aspect of the management of CKD. A principle goal of a well-planned, (very) low protein dietary regime is to decrease the accumulation of unexcreted waste products while maintaining an adequate nutritional state and improving symptoms of uraemia. This goal has been achieved by compliant CKD patients. When the diet contains less than the minimum daily requirement of 0.6 g protein/kg b.w./day, it is necessary to supply a supplement of essential amino acids or their nitrogen-free analogues (keto acids) to meet nutritional needs of CKD patients. These diets are sufficient for maintaining or improving nutritional status.

The International Advisory Board Meetings focus on identifying the risks and treatment potential for protein-restricted diets for CKD patients, especially dietary regimens supplemented with keto/amino acids.

William Mitch, Atlanta, Ga., USA

KARGER

Fax + 41 61 306 12 34
E-Mail karger@karger.ch
www.karger.com

Accessible online at:
www.karger.com/ajn

Keto Acid Therapy in CKD Patients

Epidemiology of CKD Worldwide

Hans-Jürgen Schober-Halstenberg
Berlin, Germany

The QuaSi-Niere-GmbH, Berlin, maintains the German National Registry of renal replacement therapy. Annual reports summarize the results of dialysis centre

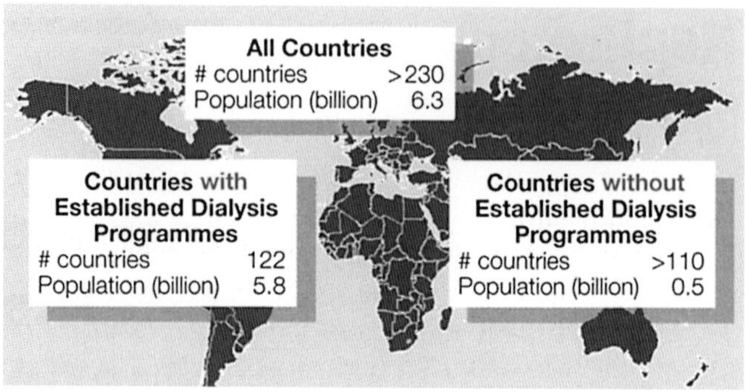

Fig. 1. ESRD population worldwide.

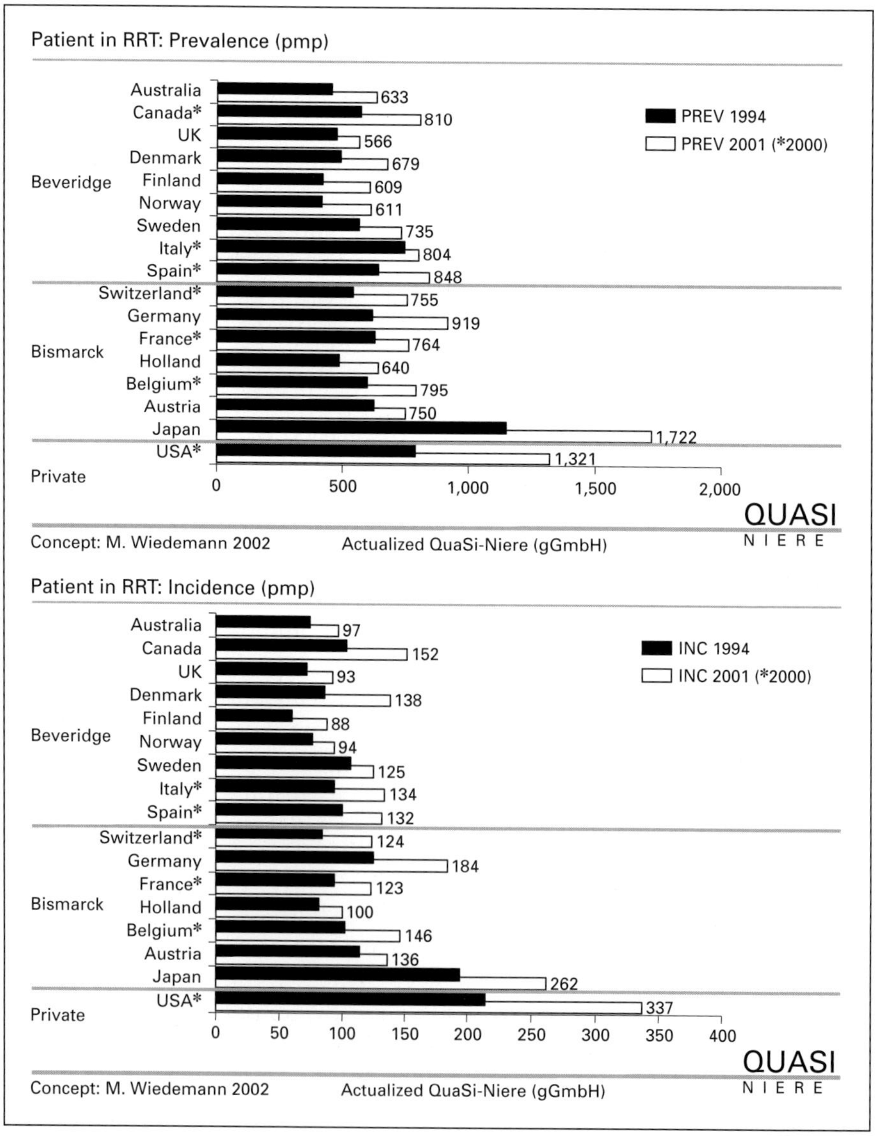

Fig. 2. Prevalence and incidence of renal replacement therapy of different countries: comparison 1984 versus 2001 (2000).

surveys and continuous patient data recording since 1996. On 31 December 2001, 1,164 facilities for dialysis and renal transplantation treatment were reported to the QuaSi-Niere-GmbH. The longitudinal data of more than 85,000 patients are available (diagnosis, modality, morbidity, follow-up).

Concerning the worldwide end-stage renal disease (ESRD) population including more than 230 countries (population: 6.3 billion), 122 countries have reported that they provide dialysis care to patients with renal failure (population: 5.8 billion) (fig. 1).

Countries where renal replacement therapy (RRT) has become standard therapy include USA, Japan, Germany, Brazil and Italy. The values for the prevalence of RRT differ between the countries (fig. 2). In 2000/2001, the highest values for the prevalence of RRT are in Japan, USA and Germany, ranging from 1,722 patients per million population (pmp) in Japan to 919 pmp in Germany, the lowest values are in UK, Finland, Norway, Australia and Netherlands (566 to 640 pmp). The same proportion can be seen regarding the incidence of RRT (fig. 2).

In general, the prevalence as well as the incidence of RRT have increased over the years from 1994 to 2000/2001 and they correlate with the wealth of the country. A comparison of the national economic strength (expressed as gross domestic product (GDP)) with the prevalence of ESRD suggests that economic factors may impose restrictions on treatment. Restriction of dialysis treatment is suggested in countries in which the gross domestic product per capita is below a limiting value. This correlation does not seem to be valid for countries in the European Union. In highly-developed countries there are three different kinds of health care models:

(1) Beveridge model: national health service (e.g. UK, Spain, Italy, Scandinavia, Canada, Australia),

(2) Private model: insurance (USA),

(3) Bismarck model: national health service plus insurance (e.g. Germany, France, Belgium, Switzerland, Netherlands, Austria, Japan).

In 2001, the expenditure for health (expressed as % GDP) ranges from 7 to 14% GDP, whereas the highest costs are in the private model (USA: 14%). In future, the total expenditure on health will increase dramatically, based on findings for the period between 1994 and 2001.

Three other aspects should be noted: (1) The increasing healthy life expectancy (in 2001 approximately 68 years for male and 72 years for female). (2) The increasing median age of patients on dialysis. (3) The exponential growth of diabetic nephropathy as a cause of ESRD.

Dietary Therapy in CKD Patients – The Current Status

William E. Mitch
Atlanta, Ga., USA

The metabolism of dietary protein results in the accumulation of waste products and ions derived from essential and non-essential amino acids in dietary protein or protein stores that are degraded. The net loss of amino acids results in an increased production of urea, and urea, like other waste products, must be eliminated via the kidneys.

A principal goal in utilizing dietary protein restriction is to decrease the accumulation of unexcreted waste products while maintaining an adequate nutritional state. This will improve the symptoms of uremia and reduce the complications of CKD, possibly even slowing the progression of renal insufficiency. There is abundant evidence that these goals can be achieved when patients are compliant with well-planned, (very) low-protein (keto/amino acid-supplemented) dietary regimens.

Notably, it has been shown that protein intake spontaneously decreases in patients with progressive CKD, but this does not represent an argument against the use of dietary protein restriction. Rather, it is a persuasive reason to restrict dietary protein intake to minimize uremic complications.

The design of a low-protein diet (0.6 g protein/kg b.w./day) or a very low protein diet (0.3 g protein/kg b.w./day) supplemented with keto amino acids requires attention to the intakes of protein, energy, vitamins and minerals. With proper supervision, such diets yield neutral nitrogen balance and are nutritionally sound. CKD patients maintain body weight (b.w.) and protein stores while being treated with these diets, in part because they can activate compensatory mechanisms that conserve protein stores in the body as long as there are no complicating diseases.

Success with dietary therapy requires periodic assessment of dietary compliance and nutritional status. There is a simple method for estimating the protein intake of CKD patients. The method is based on urea nitrogen production because nitrogen derived from the breakdown of dietary or endogenous protein is principally urea, so the sum of urea nitrogen excreted plus urea nitrogen accumulated closely parallels protein intake. In contrast, the nitrogen in urinary compounds such as creatinine, uric acid, ammonia, etc. and that in faeces (i.e. non-urea nitrogen excretion) does not vary significantly with protein intake: it averages 0.031 g nitrogen/kg ideal b.w./day. To monitor compliance with dietary protein prescription, the

24-hour urea nitrogen excretion is added to this estimate of non-urea nitrogen excretion.

Nutritional status is monitored by serial measurements of anthropometrics (especially weight), serum albumin and transferrin. Beside beneficial effects on improving symptoms of uremia and maintaining an adequate nutritional state, there is evidence that a (very) low protein diet supplemented with keto/amino acids can slow the progressive loss of kidney function. Other reports emphasize that such dietary regimen can produce a pronounced delay in time until dialysis or transplantation are required (1 year or more even when started late in the course of kidney failure).

In summary, (keto/amino acid-supplemented) protein-restricted diets should play a principal role in the treatment of patients with CKD because such a diet improves symptoms, maintains a good nutritional state, limits proteinuria and can delay the time until renal replacement therapy is needed. Despite these benefits, (keto/amino acid-supplemented) protein-restricted diets may not be offered to patients. Reasons given for avoiding this type of therapy include the difficulty in designing a low-protein diet, the difficulty in achieving compliance by the patients, the costs of keto amino acids (but these costs are below that of dialysis) and the results of the MDRD Study. This study enrolled the largest number of patients and was a trial of the influence of dietary protein restriction on progression of CKD. The effect of dietary protein restriction and blood pressure control on the progression of renal diseases was studied in a randomized fashion in 840 patients with renal failure caused by different diseases. In Study A, of 585 patients with moderate renal failure (25–55 ml/min/1.73 m^2), dietary protein was restricted to 0.58 g/kg b.w./day and did not lead to a statistically significant slowing in the rate of decline in GFR at 3 years compared to patients receiving a protein-rich diet (1.2 g/kg b.w./day). In Study B, of 255 patients with more severe renal failure (13–24 ml/min/1.73 m^2) there was a trend towards a slower decline in the renal function in a group assigned to a keto/amino acid-supplemented very low protein diet (0.28 g/kg b.w./day) compared to those who ingested a prescribed intake of 0.58 g protein/kg b.w./day. In Study B, there was no control group. Results from the MDRD Study were accepted as proof that dietary protein restriction does not slow the progression of CKD. However, there are problems with accepting this conclusion. A major problem is that the analysis of the response was based on the prescribed but not the achieved protein intake, i.e., changes in GFR were not based on what the patients ate but rather on the amount of protein the patients were told to eat. When another analysis was performed based on how much protein the patients actually ate, it was found that a decrease in protein intake did slow the loss of kidney function: a decrease in protein intake from 0.9 to 0.6 g/kg b.w./day resulted in a 33% slowing of the progression. For each 0.2 g/kg b.w./day reduction in protein intake, there was an associated 29% slower rate of loss of GFR and prolongation until dialysis was required.

In principle, protein restriction could reduce the risk of renal failure by slowing the progression of renal disease, but it also could be beneficial by ameliorating uremic symptoms. In the latter case, the dietary regime can postpone the need for dialysis without compromising the nutritional state.

Keto/Amino Acids in the Treatment of Chronic Kidney Disease Patients: 30 Years Experience in 3,000 Patients

Vladimir Teplan

Prague, Czech Republic

The long-year experiences with the use of keto/amino acids in the Institute for Clinical and Experimental Medicine, Department of Nephrology, Prague, provide a series of additional information about the metabolic consequences of such a keto/amino acid regime in chronic kidney disease patients.

Several studies have shown that adequate protein-energy nutrition and even nitrogen balance can be obtained by administering ketoanalogues of essential amino acids along with a sufficient energy intake (145 kJ/kg b.w./day). Furthermore, the minimal effective dose of ketoanalogues during long-term treatment with a standard low-protein diet has been defined as approximately 100 mg/kg b.w./day.

The evaluation of the effects of a concomitant administration of ketoanalogues and recombinant human erythropoietin (rHuEPO) on metabolic and renal parameters has shown beneficial effects on lipid metabolism (triglyceride, VLDL, IDL, LDL and Lp(a), HDL-cholesterol). Despite an initial transient decrease in the values of C_{Cr} and C_{in}, it exerts a favourable effect on the progression of renal insufficiency. Furthermore, the concomitant administration of ketoanalogues and rHuEPO results in the

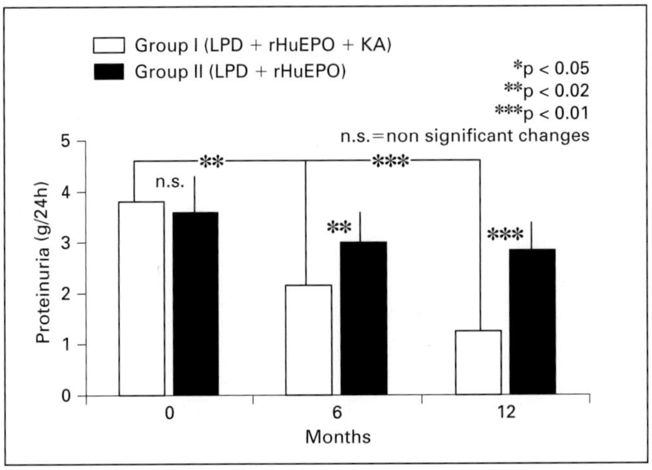

Fig. 1. Effects of a concomitant administration of ketoanalogues and recombinant human erythropoietin (rHuEPO) on proteinuria at baseline, 6 and 12 months of treatment [Teplan et al., Wien Klin Wochenschr 2001;113:17–18, 661–669].

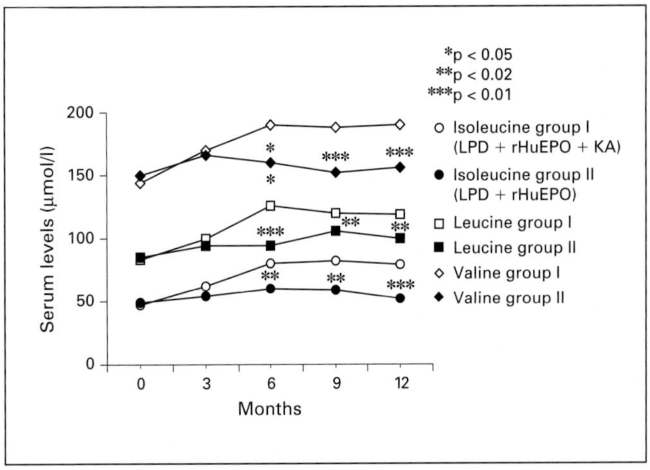

Fig. 2. Effects of a concomitant administration of ketoanalogues and recombinant human erythropoietin (rHuEPO) on serum levels of branched-chain amino acids during 12 months of treatment [Teplan et al., Wien Klin Wochenschr 2001;113:17–18, 661–669].

normalization of protein and amino acid metabolism and decrease in proteinuria (fig. 1).

Keto/amino acid regime was also associated with an increase in the serum levels of branched-chain amino acids (leucine, isoleucine and valine) (fig. 2) and a decrease in their fractional excretion as a result of a change in the tubular transport.

A multicenter study lasting several years was designed to establish whether supplementation with erythropoietin (EPO) exerts additional beneficial metabolic effects in patients with chronic kidney disease (CKD) treated with keto acids (KAs) added as a supplement to a low-protein diet (LPD: 0.6 g/kg b.w./day). This study used three therapeutic protocols: (1) EPO plus KAs plus LPD (group I), (2) EPO plus LPD (group II), and (3) LPD (group III). 186 randomly selected patients (90 men, 96 women; age: 22–78 years) with a creatinine clearance of 29.4 ± 8.2 ml/min and signs of renal anemia (hemoglobin <10.5 g/dl and hematocrit <30%) were monitored at the beginning and at every 6 months for 3 years. During the study period, the concomitant administration of the keto/amino acid regime and EPO led to a decrease in the progression of CKD (fig. 3), decrease in proteinuria, normalization of metabolic disorders as well as normalization of amino acid, protein, calcium-phosphate, carbohydrate and lipid metabolisms.

In summary, the administration of a keto/amino acid regime together with other renoprotective interventions shows numerous beneficial effects on metabolism of proteins, amino acids and lipids, delays the progression of CKD and reduces proteinuria. Such a conservative management presents an effective treatment modality for nondiabetic and diabetic CKD patients.

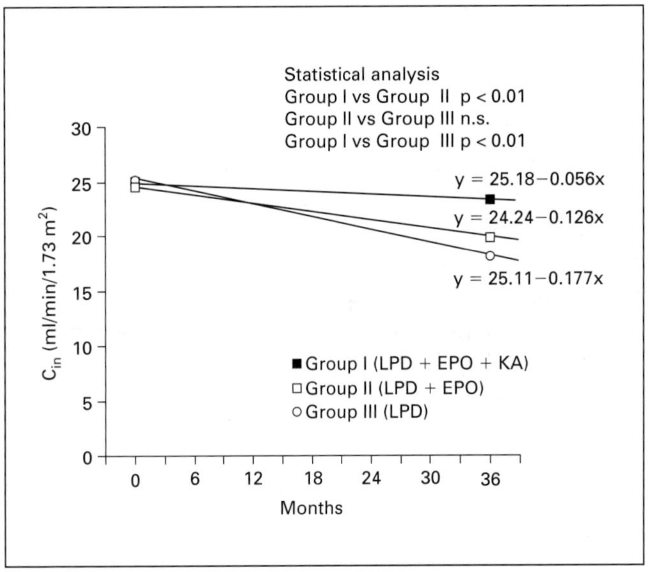

Fig. 3. Effects of a concomitant administration of ketoanalogues and recombinant human erythropoietin (rHuEPO) on serum levels of branched-chain amino acids during 12 months of treatment [Teplan et al., Am J Kidney Dis 2003;41(suppl. 1):S26–S30].

Eight Years of Ketosteril® Treatment in Hungary

Gabor Zakar
Székesfehérvár, Hungary

In 1995 an ad hoc committee of the Hungarian Nephrological Society (MANET) prepared a guideline for the keto acid treatment of predialysis and dialysis patients. On this basis the National Insurance Company (OEP) started to reimburse keto acid treatment (1 tablet Ketosteril®/5 kg b.w./day) for an initial number of 600 patients with 100% compensation. At the moment 934 patients in 59 centres use keto acids (Ketosteril®) in Hungary. Data about the compliance of such a dietary intervention show an initial dropout rate of 23%. Indications for keto acid treatment in predialysis patients are a GFR <25 ml/min/1.73 m^2, a monthly loss of GFR >0.5 ml/min on a low protein diet and/or concomitant signs of malnutrition. Indications for keto acid treatment in dialysis patients are signs of malnutrition (serum albumin <35 g/l, SGA score 'B' or <6/24) on start of dialysis and/or during dialysis.

The Hungarian Ketosteril® follow-up cohort study (1995–1997) evaluates the feasibility and effects of a low protein diet supplemented with keto acids/amino acids (KA) on the progression of chronic kidney disease (CKD) in a large group of predialysis patients and on nutritional parameters in both predialysis and dialysis patients. Predialysis (n = 181) and dialysis (n = 42) patients treated in 47 Hungarian nephrology and dialysis centres were followed during 18 months. A standardized dietary and keto/amino acid supplementation protocol was prescribed (predialysis group: 0.1 g Ketosteril®/kg b.w./day; dietary protein 0.5–0.6 g/kg b.w./day; energy 30 kcal/kg b.w./day; dialysis group: dietary protein 1.2 g/kg b.w./day, Ketosteril® and energy prescription similar to the predialysis group). In predialysis patients there was a diminution of 1/sCr equation slopes independent from the degree of renal dysfunction (sCr 201 – >600 mmol/l) (fig. 1).

Serum albumin levels below 35 g/l improved significantly during Ketosteril® supplementation on a low protein diet. In dialysis patients there was an improvement in SGA scores.

It can be concluded that in a large group of predialysis patients prescription of a low protein diet supplemented with Ketosteril® is feasible and leads to a retardation in the rate of CKD progression. Those patients require dialysis after an approximately 40% longer period than patients without this dietary intervention/medication. From the economical point of view, the yearly costs of low protein diets supplemented with keto/amino acids are approximately 1/10 of dialysis costs. Furthermore, there was an improvement in nutritional parameters in both, predialysis and dialysis patients.

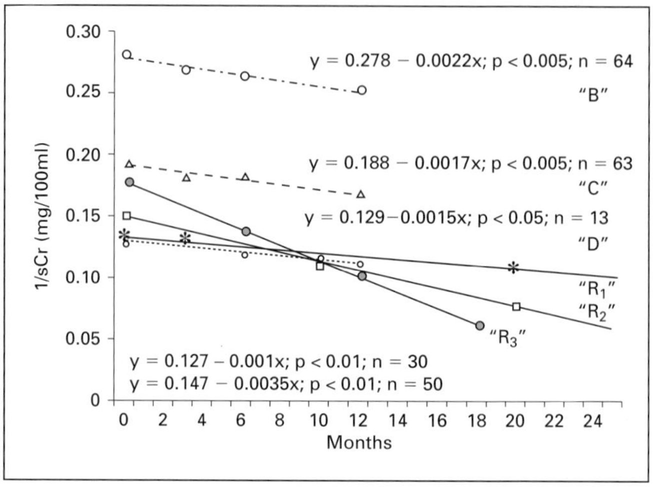

Fig. 1. Mean reciprocal serum creatinine values of KA supplemented predialysis patients. Open cycles: group 'B', sCr 201–400 mol/l, triangles: group 'C': sCr 401–600 mol/l, pentagons: group 'D', sCr 600 mol/l; line 'R_1' (asterisks): KA (keto acid-supplemented LPD [Schmicker et al., Contr Nephrol 1986;53:121–126], line 'R_2' (rectangles): EAA (essential amino acid)-supplemented LPD [Schmicker et al., Contr Nephrol 1986;53:121–126], line 'R_3' (dots) no protein restriction [Ihle et al., N Engl J Med 1989;321:1773–1777] (Zakar et al., Wien Klin Wochenschr 2001;113:17–18, 688–694).

Overview of the Uremia Program

Sergio Draibe
São Paulo, Brazil

In the Outpatient Clinic of the Nephrology Division of the Federal University of São Paulo physicians and nutritionists are enrolled in a fellowship program that enables the conservative management, including a low protein diet with or without keto/amino acid supplementation of 200–400 chronic kidney disease (CKD) patients.

At the Outpatient Clinic, experiences with protein-restricted diets include (1) low protein diet sensu latu, (2) very low protein diet supplemented with amino acids and (3) very low protein diet supplemented with Ketosteril®.

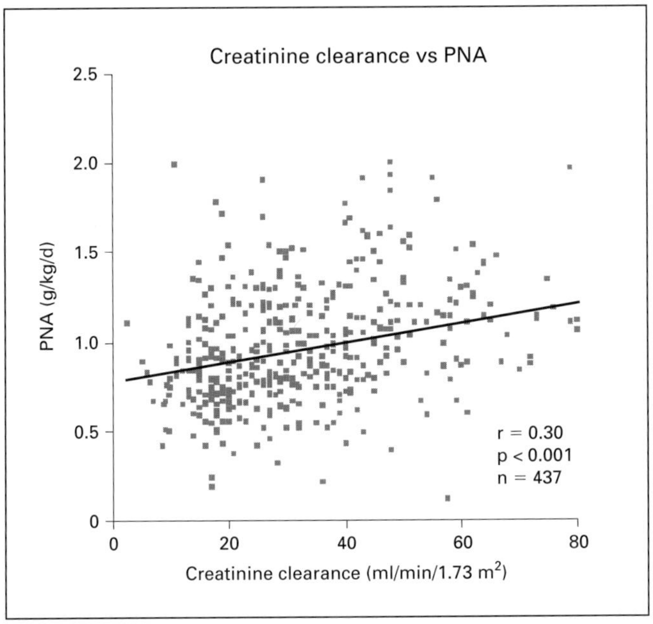

Fig. 1. Relation between creatinine clearance protein equivalent of nitrogen appearance (PNA) [Duenhas et al., European J Clin Nutr 2003;57:1473–1478].

In one recent investigation, the Outpatient Clinic analysed the spontaneous food intake and the nutrition parameters of patients with different degrees of chronic renal insufficiency at the onset of predialysis treatment. Patients were divided according to creatinine clearance (CrCl) quartiles. CrCl in the first quartile was lower than 19.9 ml/min/1.73 m^2 and in the forth one was higher than 43 ml/min/1.73 m^2. Energy intake was significantly lower in the first quartile when compared with the fourth one, while protein intake estimated by protein equivalent of nitrogen appearance was significantly lower in the first, second and third quartiles in comparison to the fourth. BMI was significantly decreased in the three lowest levels of renal functions. Compared with the fourth quartile, standard percent of midarm muscle circumference (MAMC) was lower in the second and in the third quartile. CrCl correlated directly and significantly with the protein equivalent of nitrogen appearance (fig. 1), energy intake and MAMC.

This study suggests that a spontaneous decrease in energy and protein intake as well as in anthropometric indices follows a decline in renal function in patients without previous dietary intervention.

The aim of another study was the evaluation of the efficacy and safety of very low protein diet plus essential amino acids and histidine in ESRD patients with indication to initiate dialysis therapy. The comparision of the analysed parameter at baseline and at the end of the study showed a reduction in urea concentration as well as no differences in creatinine serum concentration and creatinine clearance. Furthermore, no difference concerning the anthropometric parameters (b.w., TSF, MAMC) could be detected.

A recent study on the effects of a very low protein diet supplemented with keto/amino acids in predialysis chronic kidney disease patients has been started. This study investigates the influences of a very low protein diet supplemented with keto/amino acids (Ketosteril®) on clinical and nutritional parameters of patients with an uncomplicated advanced chronic kidney disease (CKD) (GFR <25 ml/min/1.73 m^2) in the predialysis period. At the beginning of the investigation 24 patients were assigned to a low protein diet (0.6 g protein/kg b.w./day) for at least 30 days. Afterwards, on a 4-month follow-up, 12 patients received a very low protein diet of vegetarian origin (protein: 0.3 g/kg b.w./day) supplemented with Ketosteril® (1 tablet/5 kg ideal b.w./day) (= keto acid group) and 12 patients received a low protein diet (0.6 g/kg b.w./day) of high biological value (= control group). In both groups, the prescribed energy intake was 30–35 kcal/kg b.w./day. The protein intake decreased significantly only in the keto acid group; the energy intake estimated by diaries was lower than that prescribed at the beginning of the study and did not change in both groups during the follow-up period. The nutritional state (BMI, TSF, MAMC, body fat, fat-free mass, albumin, transferrin) and renal function remained constant in both groups. Serum urea and phosphorus, and urinary phosphorus decreased significantly only in the keto acid group. The levels of serum calcium and PTH did not modify during the 4-month study period in both groups.

The initial results of this investigation confirmed that a very low protein diet supplemented with Ketosteril® maintains the nutritional status and the renal function of the patients and promoted a reduction of serum urea, serum and urinary phosphorus, constituting another therapeutic alternative for the predialysis chronic kidney disease patients.

The Pisa Experience on the Use of Keto Acids in Nephrology

Adamasco Cupisti
Pisa, Italy

Studies concerning the efficacy of protein-restricted diets have a long history, especially in Italy. The rationales for the use of keto acids on low protein/low phosphorus regimens are

(1) the control of phosphate balance, hyperphosphatemia and secondary hyperparathyroidism;

(2) the nutritional adequacy, correction of metabolic acidosis and uremic symptoms, and

(3) the retardation of progression of renal failure and the postponing of initiation of maintenance dialysis, as well as the reduction of the frequency of dialysis sessions.

The Ketodiet used at the University of Pisa contains 30–35 kcal/kg b.w./day, 65% from carbohydrates, 30% from lipids and 4% from proteins (0.3 g/kg b.w./day) supplemented with keto/amino acids (1 tablet/5 kg b.w./day), calcium carbonate (1–3 g/day) and vitamin B_{12} (1,000 U/week).

The assessment of the nutritional status is important in the management of predialysis patients, being malnutrition a major determinant of morbidity and mortality in chronic kidney disease patients.

Evidence exists that prevalence of malnutrition is largely increased when GFR <10 ml/min. Thus, in a recent study, we aimed to evaluate the factors associated with abnormal subjective global assessment (SGA) in patients with severe CKD on a low-protein diet (0.6 g protein/kg b.w./day) (LPD) or on a very-low-protein diet (0.3 g protein/kg b.w./day) supplemented with essential amino acids and keto acids (Ketodiet).

The prevalence of SGA abnormalities was higher in the patients prescribed the LPD than those prescribed the Ketodiet (45 vs. 27%, $p < 0.05$). This finding is consistent with the concept that nutritional status can be maintained better in patients eating a very-low-protein diet supplemented with essential amino acids and keto acids than in patients on standard LPD, at least in patients with severe CKD. Moreover, SGA abnormalities were associated to higher serum levels of urea and lower serum bicarbonate, at the same GFR values, suggesting that a proper dietary implementation and correction of metabolic acidosis are mandatory to reduce the risk of malnutrition.

Some skeletal muscle features were also studied in 28 non-diabetic patients with severe CKD (GFR <15 ml/min) on dietary conservative treatment. Of them, 14 were on a conventional low-protein (0.6 g/kg b.w./day) diet (LPD) and 14 were on a vegetarian very-low-protein (0.3 g/kg b.w./day) diet supplemented with essential amino acids and keto acids (Ketodiet). Three non-invasive tests investigating some skeletal muscle characteristics were performed:

(a) The myoelectrical fatigue phenomenon was studied using a surface electromyography technique that provides data on conduction velocity (CV), median frequency of power spectrum (MDF) and average rectified value (ARV) of myofibers action potential at 15 Hz and 35 Hz stimulation frequency.

(b) The muscle oxidative metabolism was studied by lactate production after aerobic exercise.

(c) The muscle strength of the legs was studied using an isokinetic exercise test performed at two different angular velocities (60° and 180°/s).

The results showed an abnormal oxidative metabolism and a reduced segmental muscle strength, whereas the surface electromyography data suggested unchanged sarcolemma excitability, normal myofiber dimension and composition of the skeletal muscle of CKD patients on dietary management. No difference was found between LPD and Ketodiet patients regarding the studied muscular parameters. As a whole, our data indicate that there are no deleterious effects of the Ketodiet regimen on skeletal muscle.

A low-protein vegetarian diet has also an anti-proteinuric effect. Thus supplementation of essential amino and keto acids could be of nutritional value in nephrotic patients, especially in the case of dietary manipulations that consist in changes in the quantity and quality of protein intake.

Another treatment opportunity for safely selected, motivated chronic kidney disease patients is the combined dietary-dialysis treatment, which includes an once-a-week hemodialysis plus very-low-protein/low-phosphorus diet supplemented with essential amino and keto acids. With this kind of treatment a nutritional adequacy can be guaranteed, the residual renal function and the diuresis volume can be preserved and the phosphate balance can be well controlled. Some favourable psychological, social and economic aspects can be taken into account as well. This combined treatment should be considered a 'gently way' of starting dialysis, and it should be reserved for selected and highly motivated patients in well-trained and motivated centers, or where dialysis facilities are lacking.

The Chronic Kidney Disease in Mexico

Rubén Darío Bonilla Aguirre
Guadalajara, Mexico

In Mexico, chronic kidney disease (CKD) is – as in the whole world – a big public health problem. About 60,000 patients are dialysed and 800,000 patients with CKD are without dialysis treatment. The treatment costs of almost 95% of the ESRD patients are covered by the social security (e.g. IMSS, SSA, ISSSTE). The highest expenses are for dialysis treatment and transplantation (approximately 90%) and only 10% of the monetary recourses are spent for predialysis treatment. In Mexico, a national program for detection and treatment of CKD (inclusive keto acid supplementation), published by the IMSS, is available.

The most important cause of CKD is long-lasting diabetes – more than 60% of the CKD patients suffer from a diabetic nephropathy.

An analysis of the experiences in the early predialytic treatment of patients with diabetic nephropathy shows that a very low protein diet (0.4 g/kg b.w./day) supplemented with keto/amino acids (1 tablet Ketosteril®/8 kg b.w./day) (Ketodiet) compared with a low protein diet (0.6 g/kg b.w./day) improves several metabolic disturbances and has a beneficial effect on the renal function.

Ketodiet regimen resulted in a decrease in serum lipid fractions (e.g. trigylcerides and cholesterol), in uric acid, glucose and phosphate as well as in an increase in serum calcium and hemoglobin. Furthermore, the Ketodiet regime preserved the renal function (analysed as creatinine clearance) for approximately 42 months, whereas a low protein diet regime resulted in a decrease in the creatinine clearance to 10 ml/min within the same period.

In Mexico, current patient groups are treated with Ketosteril®:

1 CKD secondary to diabetes mellitus
2 CKD of other etiology
3 CKD plus hepatic insufficiency
4 Children with CKD
5 Renal transplant patients and chronic rejection

In summary, the early treatment of predialysis patients with a Ketosteril® -supplemented protein-restricted diet has several benefits: it preserves renal function, it guarantees a better patient approval and, for the economical point of view, it is a cheap treatment compared to dialysis treatment and transplantation. However, more experiences with a bigger patient group and a large scientific methodology are required in order to demonstrate the effectiveness of this treatment in the early phase of illness.

Pharmacological Features of a Keto Amino Acid Therapy

Vladimir Teplan, Prague
Czech Republic

In the Czech Republic about 30,000 patients (about 3,000 patients per million inhabitants) suffer from CKD. The first sign of CKD is microalbuminuria (which can be already detected at a creatinine clearance of about 100 ml/min/1.73m^2); in contrast, proteinuria will be diagnosed in later stages (fig. 1). The most common progression-enhancing factors are hypertension, long-lasting diabetes, proteinuria, secondary hyperparathyroidism, dyslipidemia, metabolic acidosis and also dietary protein supply.

Correction measures include the control and management of blood pressure, hyperglycemia, proteinuria and a dietary management as well as the correction of several metabolic disturbances.

The keto amino acid therapy contains a dietary protein restriction as well as a supplementation of keto/amino acids essential for patients with CKD. Keto acids are the nitrogen-free analogues of amino acids, which can be converted (transaminated) in the human body into the corresponding amino acids by about 70%.

Keto acids not only substitute for their respective amino acid and maintain nitrogen balance but also exert other desirable properties:

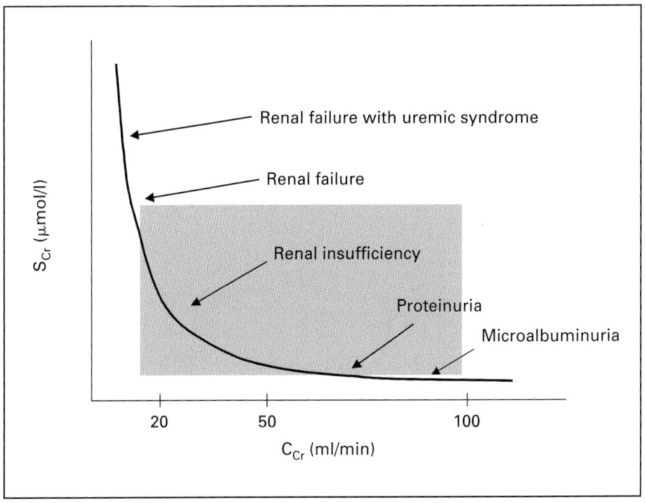

Fig. 1. Stages of chronic kidney disease depending on serum creatinine (S_{Cr}).

(1) The saving of nitrogen due to the transfer of the amino group to the keto acid is associated with a direct inhibition of ureagenesis. The inhibition is related to the increased activity of branched-chain amino acid transferase resulting in less availability of the ramified keto acid for oxidative decarboxylation.

(2) Keto acids have the ability to stimulate protein synthesis and inhibit protein degradation. Oral administration of leucine enhances protein synthesis in association with increased phosphorylation of two proteins (eukaryotic initiation factor eIF4E binding protein (4E-BP)1 and ribosomal protein S6 kinase S6K1) that control in part the step in translation initiation involving the binding of mRNA to the 40S ribosomal subunits.

(3) Administration of keto acids may lead to a partial correction of the amino acid profile in uremic patients that is also favoured by the simultaneous correction of metabolic acidosis due to the reduced alimentary intake of sulphur-containing amino acids. In addition, the decrease in urinary protein excretion due to amino/keto acid-supplemented protein-restricted diets contributes to the rise in serum albumin and the maintenance of various indices of nutritional status within the normal range. Compared to other amino acids, keto acids lack a stimulating effect on hyperfiltration of the kidney. Following the supply of keto acids of branched-chain amino acids (BCAA) during a protein-restricted diet, the pancreatic glucagon stimulation and the subsequent glucagon-induced hepatic cAMP secretion that is typical for amino acids is missing.

(4) Metabolic acidosis results from impaired excretion of hydrogen ions. A large proportion of the hydrogen ions come from the metabolism of sulphur-containing amino acids. This acidosis has several deleterious effects, namely on protein metabolism, glucose tolerance and bone metabolism. Only strict reduction or suppression of protein of animal origin is susceptible to correct metabolic acidosis. Since metabolic acidosis increases the degradation of branched-chain amino acids and protein catabolism, and suppresses albumin synthesis, the control of this disorder is especially important in patients with a reduced protein intake.

(5) Protein-restricted diets which do not contain proteins of animal origin reduce phosphorus intake, and the presence of calcium (calcium salts of the keto-analogues in Ketosteril®) has additional beneficial effects on the disturbed calcium/phosphate metabolism and secondary hyperparathyroidism.

(6) Keto/amino acid therapy is able to improve most of the disturbances in carbohydrate metabolism observed in uremia. Beneficial effects include the improvement in tissue sensitivity to insulin, reduction in circulating insulin levels in relation to an increase in the metabolic clearance rate of insulin, and improved inhibitory action of insulin on endogenous glucose production. The lowering of insulin resistance, reduction of hyperinsulinemia and increase in energy production rate in patients on a keto/amino acid therapy make it a therapeutic arm remarkably well adapted for the treatment of uremic patients, especially the growing group of obese non-insulin-dependent diabetics with CKD.

(7) Keto/amino acid therapy has beneficial effects on correction of lipid disorders, especially with respect to an decrease in triglyceride levels and an increase in HDL-cholesterol levels. These results are important because of the accelerated atherosclerosis commonly seen in uremia.

Dietary regime, used in the Institute for Clinical and Experimental Medicine, Department of Nephrology, Prague, contains 0.6 g protein, 1.3 g lipids, 4.9 g carbohydrate and 140 kJ energy/kg b.w./day supplemented with 100 mg Ketosteril®/kg b.w./day. Besides a sufficient energy intake and the amount of protein intake also the ratio of animal/vegetable protein (preferentially 1:1) seems to be important in low protein diets supplemented with Ketosteril®. In Czech Republic, many patients do not accept a strict very low protein diet (0.3 g protein/kg b.w./day) supplemented with Ketosteril®; it is mainly composed of vegetarian food.

Some important contra-indications for the intake of keto acids are an inadequate caloric intake, severe therapy-resistant arterial hypertension and a creatinine clearance lower than 5 ml/min/1.73 m^2.

Other possible indications for a keto acid therapy is its use in dialysis patients as a strategy to reduce the frequency of dialysis. In dialysis a supplementation with keto/amino acids has the aim of phosphate binding as well as improvement of the nutritional status and extention of the survival during dialysis.

Another opportunity of treatment is the infrequent dialysis. Generally, the treatment of patients with end-stage renal failure is based on the maintenance hemodialysis 3 times a week and a free diet with the only restriction being the intake of potassium, sodium and water. By adding both the detoxifying effects of dialysis and a keto/amino acid therapy, the residual renal function might be maintained and the frequency of dialysis sessions reduced. However, this treatment option is only for highly educated and motivated patients, and as noted, the aim is to save residual kidney function, to reduce the number of dialysis sessions, and to increase the quality of life by creating more freedom for working and travelling.

Nephrology in China

Shanyan Lin
Shanghai, China

China's population is about 1.259 billion. Unfortunately, in China no exact data of the nation-wide incidence of end-stage renal disease are available. As calculated from a sample from Shanghai about 18 million patients should suffer from chronic kidney disease (CKD) in China. The annual incidence rate of ESRD in Shanghai was 122/million population in 2000 and 174/million population in 2002. Due to the incomplete individual reports in different areas of China, the figures vary from 95 to 185/million population. About 80,000–100,000 patients are currently on dialysis and additionally 100,000 new ESRD patients are present each year. During the last years, there is a tremendous increase in dialysis treatment (e.g. 34,250 in 1999 versus 46,796 in 2000). Most of the dialysis patients receive a hemodialysis treatment (approximately 45%); the costs of hemodialysis (including an EPO therapy) are about 6,202–11,669 USD/person/year.

Diabetic nephropathy, as a consequence of a long-lasting diabetes, becomes more important in China. Its percentage increased from 3% in the 80s to 10–20% nowadays; however, there are differences in specific areas of China.

In China, low-protein diets are well known but are only used as an alternative to dialysis in severe CKD (especially if the patients are unable or unwilling to be dialysed). Since 1992, Ketosteril® has been introduced in China and several studies have been performed on the influence of keto/amino acids on the progression of CKD, nutritional aspects, secondary hyperparathyroidism and metabolic acidosis.

The Department of Nephrology at the Ruijin Hospital, Shanghai, investigated the effect of a low protein diet supplemented with keto/amino acids in CKD patients. This dietary regime improved metabolic acidosis and attenuated elevated cortisone levels in those patients.

Aspects favouring the future use of low protein diets supplemented with keto/amino acids in China are the disproportional force of dialysis facilities, the cultural background (dependency and hospitality in connection with dialysis are unpopular, furthermore the dialysis is seen as a final measure without any hope) and the traditional Chinese diet (the performance of a low protein diet is not that difficult).

In future, some important points have to be clarified, like the application of a low protein diet supplemented with keto/amino acids in proteinuric patients, in diabetic nephropathy and in dialysis (hemodialysis/peritoneal dialysis). Additionally, guidelines should be developed concerning the allowed protein intake in different stages of CKD and specific menu plans should be created in order to achieve a higher patient compliance. Furthermore, pharmaco-economical data should be drawn up, in order to convince nephrologists of the use of low protein diets supplemented with keto/amino acids from the economical point of view, too.

Are Supplemented Low-Protein Diets Nutritionally Safe?

Michel Aparicio
Bordeaux, France

Concerns have been raised that dietary protein restriction and more specifically supplemented very low protein diets (SVLPD) could induce malnutrition in patients in the predialysis phase of chronic kidney disease (CKD), whose nutritional status may already be altered by spontaneous decreases in energy and protein intakes. Because malnutrition increases morbidity and mortality in dialysis patients, the use of SVLPD in predialysis phase could have adverse effects on the outcome of patients on renal replacement therapy.

A lot of studies have shown that a metabolic adaptation to dietary protein restriction occurs in both healthy subjects as well as in patients with an uncomplicated chronic kidney disease. Due to this, an adequate nitrogen balance can be achieved by the long-term administration of a SVLPD. There is abundant evidence that patients following a SVLPD properly are able to maintain normal serum proteins and anthropometric indices during long-term. However, it has to take into consideration that in both, subjects with normal renal function and patients with chronic kidney disease, an initial weight loss is observed when they are shifted to a reduced protein diet. This decrease in body weight (b.w.) is accounted by loss of muscle protein. Nitrogen losses are slowly adjusted for resulting in a transient negative nitrogen balance which requires approximately 90 days to reach complete equilibrium.

In a retrospective study, performed in Bordeaux from 1985 to 1997, the influence of a SVLPD providing 0.3 g protein, 35 kcal and 5–7 mg inorganic phosphorus/kg b.w./day supplemented with Ketosteril® on the clinical outcome and nutritional status of 239 patients with advanced CKD during predialysis period and their evolu-

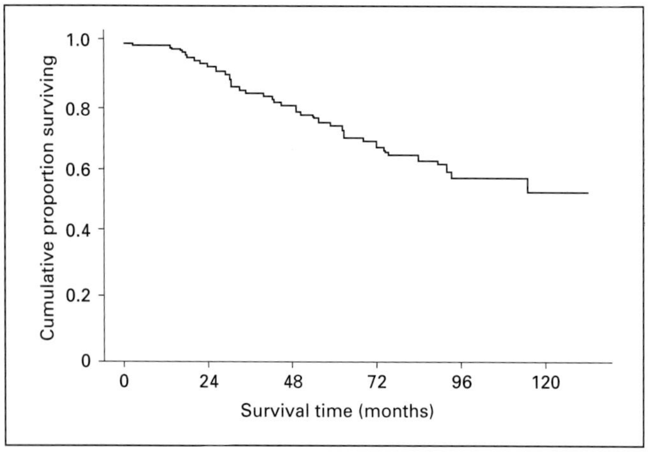

Fig. 1. Survival curve of the 165 patients treated by hemodialysis after cessation of SVLPD [Aparicio et al., J Am Soc Nephrol 2000;11:708–711].

tion after initiation of renal replacement therapy was evaluated.

During SVLPD nutritional indices like body mass index and serum albumin concentration remained unchanged overall. 20 patients discontinued this nutritional intervention and 14 patients died during SVLPD, but the death was unrelated to nutritional parameters. Hemodialysis was initiated after 29.8 ± 23.1 months on SVLPD in 165 patients at a mean GFR of 5.8 ± 1.5 ml/min. The general recommendation for the initiation of renal replacement therapy is GFR at 10.5 ml/min. From the economical point of view, the deferment of the initiation of hemodialysis (mean time interval between GFR at 10.5 ml/min and initiation of dialysis: 18.6 ± 13.2 months) saved costs up to 10,000,000 USD. During an average of 54 months on hemodialysis, the mortality was low (2.4% after 1 year) (fig. 1) and correlated to age only, not to nutritional parameters observed at the end of SVLPD. Similar results were obtained in 66 transplanted patients.

It can be concluded that a SVLPD can be safely used in selected and carefully followed-up patients with CKD even in potential catabolic situations (nephrotic syndrome, diabetic nephropathy, chronic renal rejection) without adverse effects on the clinical and nutritional status. Due to preservation of nutritional status and correction of uremic symptoms, the initiation of dialysis was substantially deferred in these patients. Furthermore, the outcome of patients on renal replacement therapy is not affected by prior treatment with SVLPD during the predialysis phase of chronic kidney disease.

Consensus
Keto Acid Therapy in CKD Patients

- A well-planned keto/amino acid-supplemented protein-restricted diet therapy as part of a treatment program
  - is safe, does not induce malnutrition and can improve metabolic abnormalities associated with renal insufficiency
  - may slow progression and will delay the time until dialysis is required to treat uremic symptoms
- A team approach between all disciplines involved (doctors/dieticians/nutritionists) is needed
- A keto/amino acid-supplemented protein-restricted diet is a cost-effective treatment therapy, and can improve the quality of life of patients in predialysis stage
- Specific international guidelines and recommendations for keto/amino acid-supplemented protein-restricted diets are specified:
  - the daily protein intake at a low-protein diet supplemented with keto acids should not exceed 0.6 g/kg b.w./day, optimal protein intake is 0.3–0.4 g/kg b.w./day
  - the recommended dosage of keto/amino acids (Ketosteril®) is 0.1 g/kg b.w./day
  - a daily energy intake of 35 kcal/kg b.w./day should be recommended
  - a low-protein diet (0.6 g protein/kg b.w./day) is indicated at a creatinine clearance of 50 ml/min/1.73 m^2, a ketodiet at a creatinine clearance of 20–25 ml/min/1.73 m^2 (however, these recommendations can be impractical in countries with different guidelines)
  - in the first 3 months after the beginning of a (very) low-protein diet supplemented with keto/amino acids (Ketosteril®) the control examinations should be recommended monthly, afterwards the intervals between the control examinations could be 2–3 months
  - the following parameters should be measured at the control examinations: 24-hour urea nitrogen, body weight, electrolytes, calcium, phosphate, PTH, serum creatinine, creatinine clearance, acid-base balance (Atrup), bicarbonate, blood counts, hemoglobin, lipids, glycaemia, transferrin (only at the beginning)
  - vitamins and iron are important supplements of a low-protein diet
  - the phosphorus intake should be 5–7 mg/kg b.w./day (500 to not more than 800 mg/day)
  - the daily salt intake should be in the range of 100 mmol sodium chloride, especially in patients with hypertension or other signs of extracellular volume overload
- Parameters for clinical studies should be agreed on

Keto Acid Therapy for Patients with Diabetic Nephropathy

Risk of Developing ESRD in Patients with Diabetic Nephropathy – Lessons from the USA

William E. Mitch
Atlanta, Ga., USA

Principal metabolic disturbances occurring in CKD patients or during uremia are all related to the accumulation of unexcreted metabolic products, which in turn arise mainly from dietary protein. Additionally, these problems are related to the progressive loss of kidney function and to the development of progressive cardiovascular disease.

In 2000, the global burden of diabetes, as the most important single course of kidney disease, was estimated world-wide of about 154 million people. For 2030 a number of 370 million is calculated, showing a significant increase in Asia and Latin America. Due to the increasing number of diabetes, connected with complications such as kidney disease, there will be no possibility that all these patients could be dialysed. Therefore, there is a real need of actions in order to intervene the development to the stage of final kidney failure.

One potential explanation for the increasing incidence of diabetes is the observed obesity associated with the occurrence of type II diabetes. In turn, these patients develop kidney failure in exactly the same fashion as people with type I diabetes.

One of the most important things that are to remember is that hypertension and diabetes go hand in hand. More than 70% of patients with type I and 90% with type II diabetes and kidney disease are hypertensive. Furthermore, 40% of patients are hypertensive before kidney disease is recognized.

Due to the fact that progression of kidney disease is directly related to blood pressure, a blood pressure of ≤130/80 mmHg in diabetes or CKD patients is recommended in order to minimize the loss of kidney function. Control of hypertension can be achieved by the use of angiotensin converting enzyme inhibitors (ACEi) or angiotensin receptor blockers. Such long-term treatment in type I and II diabetic patients with nephropathy will increase the time to first event and decrease the incidence of doubling sCr (by 48% in type I, 25% in type II) and end stage renal disease (ESRD) or death (by 50% in type I, 20% in type II). Furthermore, proteinuria and the rate of decline in renal function can be reduced – and this largely independent of the achieved blood pressure.

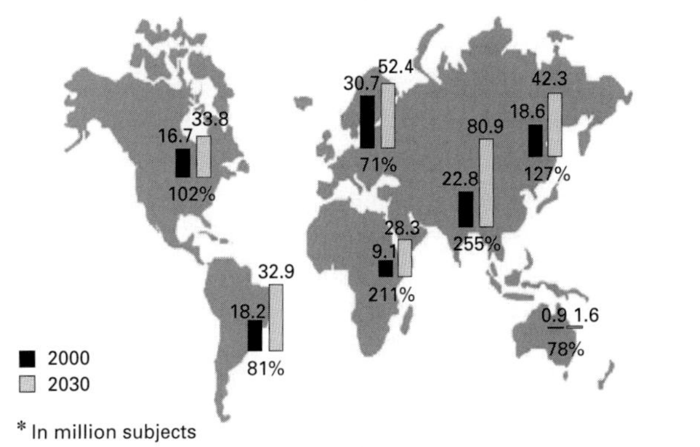

* In million subjects

	World	Developed	Developing
2000	154 m	55 m	99 m
2030	370 m	84 m	286 m

WHO, March 2003

Fig. 1. The global burden of diabetes (2000–2030).

Another strategy is a dietary intervention, namely protein restriction (0.6 protein/kg b.w./day). Meta-analysis as well as clinical studies with patients on a low protein diet, who are either diabetic or non-diabetic, shows a risk reduction for dialysis or death by 23 up to 46%. It is very clear that major problems in terms of treating hypertension is salt accumulation and very high protein diets are automatically associated with a high dietary salt intake. Therefore, hypertension becomes more and more difficult to control and low protein diets are recommended in terms of decreasing salt intake.

Proteinuria is the most common course of ESRD at least in Western countries. Once patients with type II diabetes and nephropathy develop severe proteinuria (≥0.5 g/day) the survival of the kidney averages only 3 years. Therefore, screenings of blood pressure, microalbuminuria and proteinuria that in diabetes (type I and II) are the very first signs of kidney disease are recommended as soon as the diagnosis of diabetes was made.

Several longitudinal studies with non-diabetic and diabetic patients show a direct relation between proteinuria and an increased risk of cardiovascular diseases (Framingham Study, Normal/Hypertensive Men, 10-Year Report and 5-Year Report), which is per se higher in patients even with mild renal insufficiency.

Beside control of blood pressure in type II diabetic patients with nephropathy, proteinuria, degree of renal failure, serum albumin, and hemoglobin levels are independent risk factors that predict renal outcomes. The level of proteinuria proved to be the strongest and most consistent risk factor for progressive kidney injury the basal level of proteinuria is also associated with composite renal outcome or ESRD as well as cardiovascular events in diabetic patients. Thus, one goal of treating CKD patients should be to monitor the degree of proteinuria and use therapy to reduce proteinuria.

Dietary intervention in form of a low protein-keto acid diet can suppress proteinuria without interfering with metabolic control of type II diabetic patients. After 6 months on a low protein-keto acid diet, urinary albuminuria decreased significantly; the most important observation is that a low protein diet decreased urinary albuminuria by 17% and ACEi alone decreased urinary albuminuria by 19% – but combining ACEi and low protein diet decreased urinary albuminuria by 63%.

In summary, an effective reduction of urinary albuminuria/proteinuria can reduce the risk of doubling serum creatinine, ESRD or death or/and reducing the risk of having a stroke, heart attack and congestive heart failure. Furthermore, dietary interventions such as low protein-keto acid diets can be considered as a safe therapy.

Standards of Care for Diabetic Nephropathy

Vladimir Teplan

Prague, Czech Republic

There are currently more than 117 million people with diabetes worldwide. WHO figures estimate that this will rise to 300 million in 2025. Diabetes is the fourth main course of death in most developed countries. It is estimated that diabetes accounts for 5–10% of the nation's health budget. The estimated diabetes prevalence varies between different countries (5 to 20%), but an increase in all countries is assumed within the next 20 years.

The incidence of patients with end-stage renal disease (ESRD) and type II diabetes has been increased tremendously over the past few decades. The prevalence of renal failure in diabetic patients (type I and II) is around 45–60% after 5 years. Concerning signs of diabetic nephropathy, one of the most important complications are rising urinary albumin and protein excretion, rising blood pressure, and declining kidney function. Diabetic nephropathy is also associated with an increased risk of cardiovascular disease, retinopathy, and neuropathy. Risk factors for the development of diabetic nephropathy are duration of diabetes, familiar and ethnic factors, hyperglycemia, high blood pressure, dyslipidemia, proteinuria and smoking. Especially, proteinuria is not only a marker of damage, but is also a risk factor that accelerates the rate of loss of kidney function. The prevalence of proteinuria in diabetic patients (type I and II) is around 53–75% after 25 years and is known as a sign/symptom of the fast decline of residual function.

In the context of an appropriate management of diabetic nephropathy, it is very important to detect the disease in time (at beginning of microalbuminuria). Unfortunately, many patients with diabetes are referred late to nephrologists. Consequences of late referral include poorer status upon referral, higher rates of hospitalisation and higher costs, and even increased mortality. Diabetic patients with ESRD have a high cardiovascular morbidity and mortality on dialysis, shown by a prospective study in 35 dialysis centres in Germany (1985–1994). Hereby type II diabetic patients had a lower mean survival time than type I diabetics.

In diabetics with CKD, the pathological effects of oxygen radicals can contribute to the morbidity and mortality of these patients. Hyperglycemia induces mitochondrial superoxide production, increases oxidative stress, and leads to activation of the acute-phase response. Hyperglycemia, impaired renal function, and uremia cause inflammatory and oxidative processes. Advanced oxidation protein products and advanced glycation end products are formed, leading to subsequent cytokine release. This promotes alterations in lipoprotein metabolism, composition, and function. These changes result in a highly atherogenic environment, perpetuating the vicious cycle of accelerated atherogenesis. The terminal pathway is an elevation of C-reactive protein (CRP), a biomarker of both overall and cardiovascular outcome.

Additionally, it is obvious that progressive renal failure in hypertension is linked to insulin resistance/hyperinsulinemia. The flow of substrates, hormones, and cytokines from visceral fat to skeletal muscle and endothelial cells, along with some genetic abnormalities and obesity, may play a role in establishing these shared metabolic and vascular derangements. Substantial clinical and experimental evidence suggests that both diabetes and insulin resistance cause a combination of endothelial dysfunctions. Endothelial dysfunctions that have been described include decreased endothelium-dependent vasorelaxation, vascular permeability, and the altered production of a variety of vasoactive substances, which affect coagulation, extracellular matrix homeostasis, and smooth muscle physiology. The primary mechanisms that contribute to these endothelial dysfunctions in diabetes appear to involve the activation of protein kinase C (PKC) pathways, increased non-enzymatic glycation, increased oxidative stress, and reduced endothelial insulin action. In addition, many of the adverse effects associated with hyperglycemia and insulin resistance are mediated and amplified by potent growth factors and peptides including transforming growth factor-β, platelet-derived growth factor-β, vascular endothelial growth factor, leptin, and angiotensin II. Especially, transforming growth factor-β1 (TGF-β1) affects extracellular matrix accumulation. It plays a role in thickening of peripheral basement membranes and expansion of the mesangium in several renal diseases. Furthermore, angiotensin II has several hemodynamic (e.g. systemic hypertension, increased glomerular capillary pressure and permeability, mesangial cell contraction leading to reduction in filtration surface area) and non-hemodynamic effects (e.g. induction of renal hypertrophy and cell proliferation, stimulation of cytokine and superoxide production, stimulation of extracellular matrix synthesis) contributing to the progression of kidney failure.

These observations have led to recommendations for the management of renal risk factors in people with diabetes/diabetic nephropathy (see table).

Risk factor	Treatment	Result of treatment
Hyperglycemia	HbA1c < 5–7% Drugs: insulin, oral hypoglycemic agent Lifestyle modification	Prevent appearance of albuminuria, may delay progression of nephropathy
High blood pressure	Systolic blood pressure: < 120/125 mmHg Diastolic blood pressure: < 75 mmHg Drugs: ACE inhibitors, angiotensin receptor antagonists, non-dihydropyridinic calcium blockers, beta blockers Lifestyle modification: salt restriction, exercise, loss of excess weight	Prevent diabetic nephropathy, delay progression
Dyslipidemia	LDL-Cholesterol < 115 mg/dl Drugs: statins, fibrates (caution if renal failure) Lifestyle modification	May delay progression of nephropathy
Albuminuria/ proteinuria	Drugs: ACE inhibitors, angiotensin receptor antagonists	Delay the progression of nephropathy
High intake of protein	< 0.8–0.6 g protein/kg b.w./day (plus keto acids) Reduction of protein intake depending on residual renal function In case of proteinuria: increase in protein intake according to the urinary losses	Delay the progression of nephropathy
Smoking	Stop smoking	

Studies concerning the efficacy of dietary protein restriction involving patients with diabetes and nephropathy showed that, as compared with a high intake of protein and phosphorus, the restriction of protein and phosphorus (0.6 g protein/kg b.w./day and 500–1,000 mg phosphorus/day) reduced the rate of fall of GFR and lowered blood pressure.

The Institute for Clinical and Experimental Medicine, Department of Nephrology, Prague, analysed data obtained from a prospective long-term randomized multicentric study designed to evaluate the effect of concomitant administration of keto/amino acids (KA) and ACE inhibitors (ACEi) on proteinuria and aminoaciduria in CKD patients with diabetic nephropathy assigned to a low-protein diet (LPD). The study was designed to monitor, over a 12-month period, a total of 50 patients randomized into group I (25 patients) receiving LPD (0.6 g protein/kg b.w./day), keto acids (100 mg/kg b.w./day), ACEi (perindopril 4 mg/day) and group II (25 patients) given LPD and ACEi in equal doses. The comparison of the two groups showed additional beneficial effects of combining keto/amino acid regime and ACEi therapy: there was a significant decrease in proteinuria and in progression of CKD (fig. 1), normalization of the lipid metabolism as well as an improvement of inflammatory parameters (free radicals, CRP, TGF-β, P-selectin) (fig. 2).

Due to the fact that obesity is classified as a major risk factor on the progression of CKD, a long-term prospective randomised placebo-controlled study was designed to monitor metabolic status, nutrition and progression of renal failure in obese CKD patients using two protocols: (A) low protein diet with 0.6 g protein and 30 kcal/kg b.w./day (LPD) with keto acids (KA) 100 mg/kg b.w./day (group I, 34 patients), and (B) LPD with placebo (group II, 32 patients). A total of 66 CKD patients (30 men, 36 women, aged 26–78 years, Ccr 30–48 ml/min/1.73 m^2) with BMI ≥ 30 kg/m^2 were monitored at beginning and at every 6 months for 3 years. During follow-up period decrease of GFR measured as creatinine and inulin clearances was lower in group I ($p < 0.01$). At the same time, a significant increase in serum branched-chain amino acids (BCAA), albumin, transferrin (fig. 3) and soluble leptin receptor were found in group I (all $p < 0.01$).

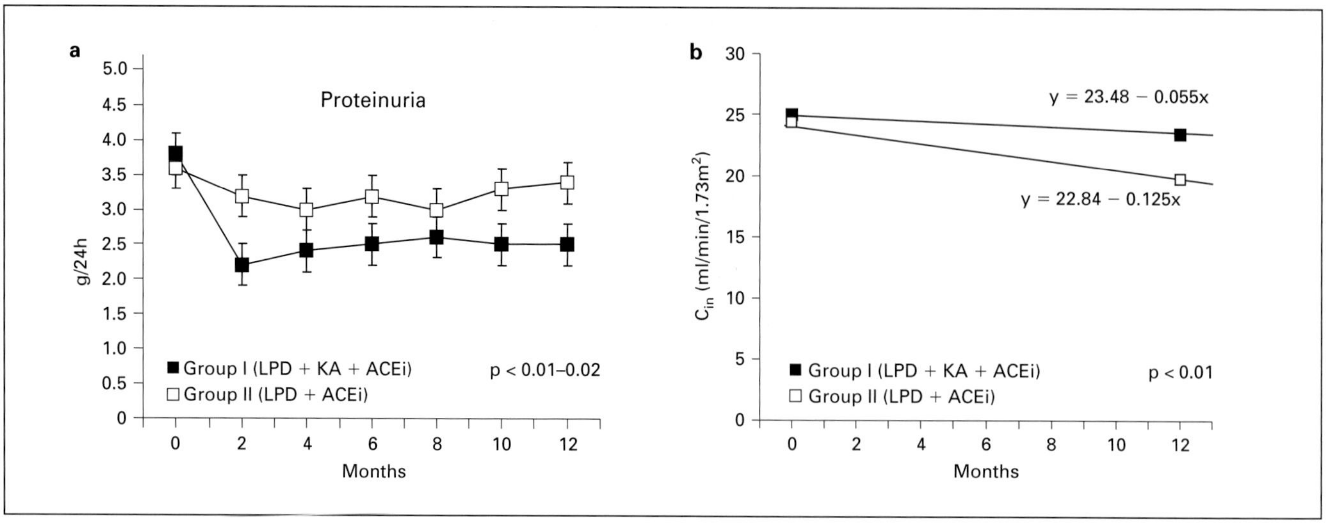

1

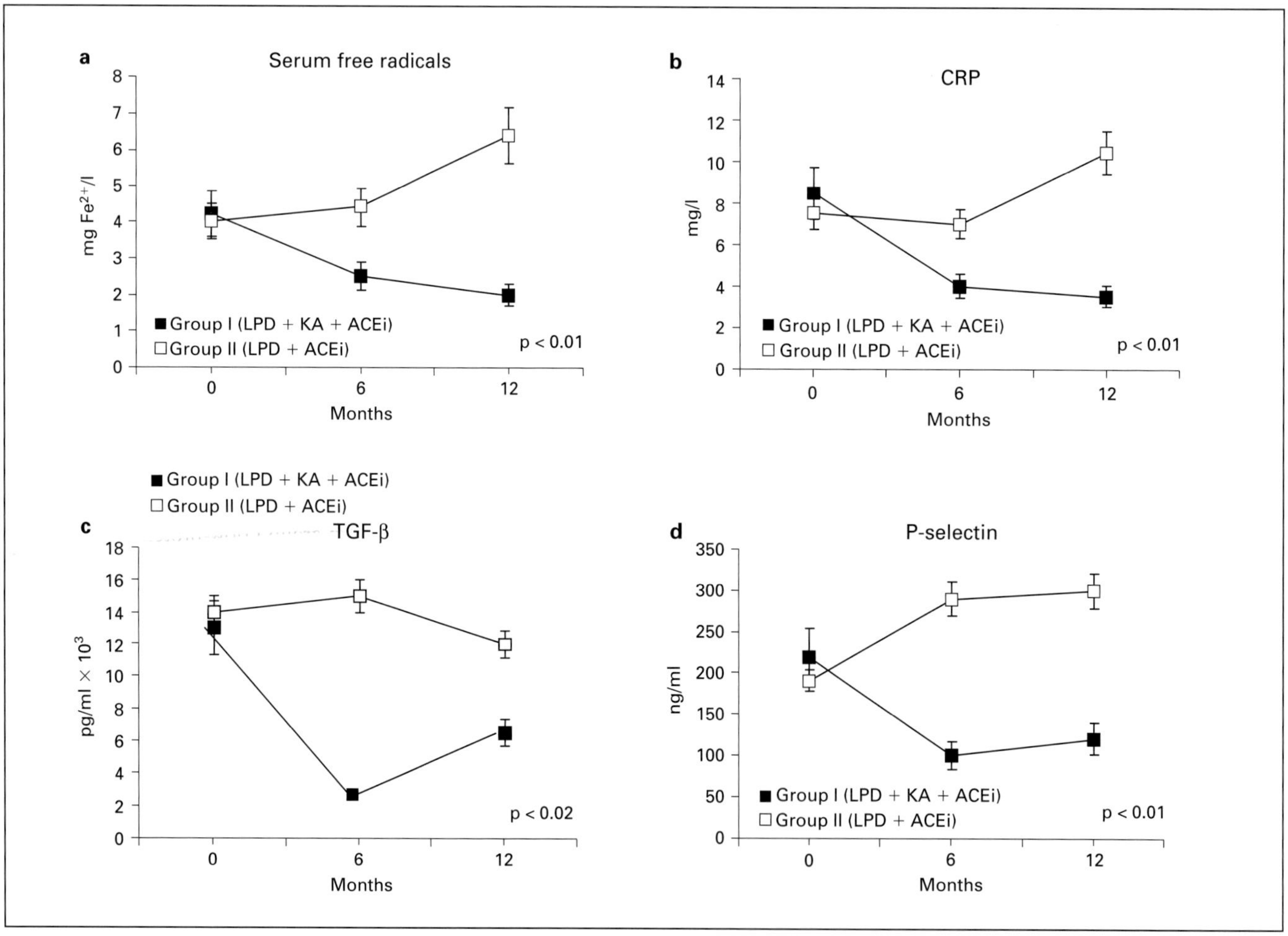

2

Fig. 1. Proteinuria and glomerular filtration by clearance of inulin in group I (low-protein diet (LPD) + keto acids (KA) + ACE inhibitor (ACEi)) and group II (low-protein diet (LPD) + ACE inhibitor (ACEi)) [Teplan et al., Klin Biochem Met 2003;2:70–73].

Fig. 2. Inflammatory parameters (free radicals, CRP, TGF-β, P-selectin) in group I (low-protein diet (LPD) + keto acids (KA) + ACE inhibitor (ACEi)) and group II (low-protein diet (LPD) + ACE inhibitor (ACEi)) [Teplan et al., Klin Biochem Met 2003;2:70–73].

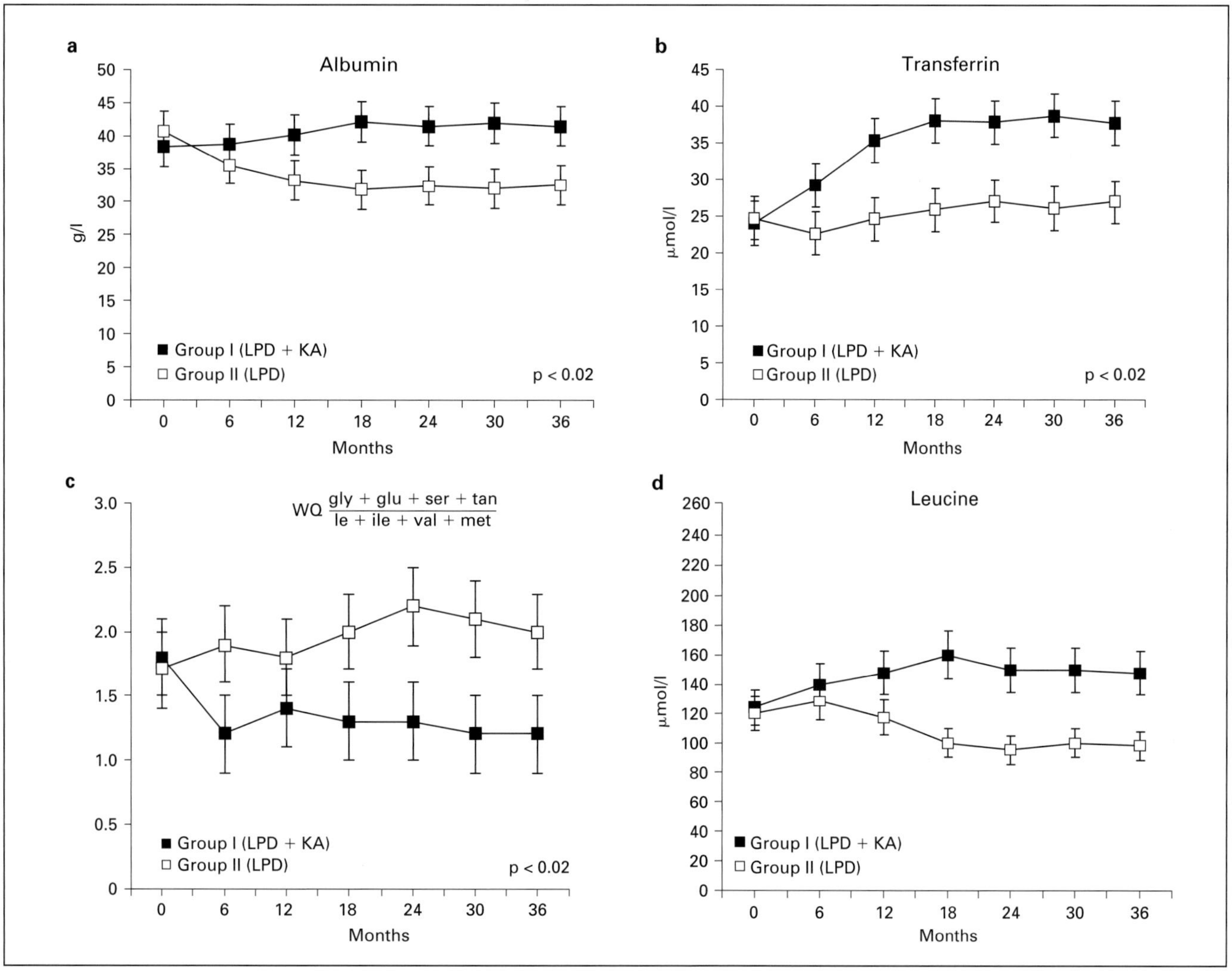

Fig. 3. Changes in albumin, transferrin and serum amino acid concentrations in group I (low-protein diet (LPD) + keto acids (KA)) and group II (low-protein diet (LPD) [Teplan et al. 2004, International Congress on Nutrition and Metabolism in Renal Disease, Italy].

In addition, significant decrease were also seen in BMI and fat in muscles, CRP, TGF-β, P- and E-selectin, ICAM I, ET I, leptin, homocysteine, proteinuria, serum triglycerides, renal fractional leucine excretion and ROS ($p < 0.01–0.02$). Obese CKD patients did no differ genetically from the Czech population (MONICA Project). Apo E isoforms and ACE polymorphism did not differ significantly. Comparing to placebo group II, co-administration of LPD with KA thus constitutes an effective alternative in management of conservative treatment in obese CKD patients delaying in follow-up period progression of renal failure with corrected metabolic parameters.

Place of Dietary Protein Restriction in the Treatment of Diabetic Nephropathy

Michel Aparicio

Bordeaux, France

A worldwide epidemic of renal failure from diabetic nephropathy is in progress. It is closely related to the rapidly growing numbers of individuals with type II diabetes. Diabetic nephropathy has become the single most important cause of end-stage renal disease. High calorie supply, sedentariness and increased aging of society favor the increased prevalence of type II diabetes. The main factors of development and progression of diabetic nephropathy are hyperglycemia, hypertension, genetic predisposition, dyslipidemia, smoking and the amount of dietary protein intake.

The efficacy of anti-hypertensive therapy and treatment of coronary heart disease allows more time to develop ESRD that is in fact – in diabetic patients – a disease of medical progress.

As diet may be related to diabetic complications, nutritional intake was analyzed in the EURODIAB IDDM Complications Study. The aims of this study were to investigate current nutrient intakes in comparison to recommended levels in 2,868 IDDM patients from 30 centers in 16 countries throughout Europe. Mean energy intake for all patients was 2,390 ± 707 kcal/day. Mean protein intake was 17.6% (1.5 ± 0.5 g/kg b.w./day), carbohydrate intake was 43% and total fat contributed 38% of energy, with 14% from saturated fat. More than 20% of patients had a higher protein intake than 20% of energy. Due to the fact that albumin excretion rate (associated with hypertension and/or poor diabetic control) significantly correlates to the intake of protein, this data clearly indicate current problems.

Nutritional recommendations of the American Diabetes Association (2001) are 50–55% of total energy intake as carbohydrates, 30–35% as fat and 10–20% as protein (both animal and vegetable sources). According to the European Association for the Study of Diabetes and the American Diabetes Association, patients with incipient or manifest nephropathy should be advised to reduce their protein intake to 0.7 to 0.9 g protein/kg b.w./day and to substitute vegetable protein for protein from animal sources which reduces intakes of total fat and saturated fatty acids.

The reduction of dietary protein intake in diabetic patients raises two potential problems:

(1) A nutritional problem: as insulin is an anabolic hormone, there is an increased risk of malnutrition related to insulinopenia (type I diabetes) or to insulin resistance (type II diabetes). Moreover, in diabetic (as in non-diabetic) patients, low-protein diet is accompanied by an increase in the energy production rate.

(2) A metabolic problem: the increased quantities of carbohydrates necessary to maintain a satisfactory energy intake during protein-restricted diets might make the control of blood glucose levels more difficult.

Arguments against these fears are that – regardless of renal function – an adaptation to dietary protein restriction occurs, defined as decrease of essential amino acid oxidation, inhibition of postprandial degradation and with feeding, less increase in protein synthesis. In diabetic patients, these factors of adaptation may be affected by the degree of metabolic control.

Different long-term studies with insulin-dependent (IDDM) and non-insulin-dependent diabetes mellitus (NIDDM) patients with progressive diabetic nephropathy on low protein diets indicated that anthropometrics, serum albumin, and body weight were comparable in patients on a low protein diet and on a usual protein diet. Of course, according to short-term and mid-term studies, nitrogen balances remained negative throughout the period of protein restriction. But it is already known that a new equilibrium after changing protein intake can only be achieved after 3 months. After adaptation to a low protein diet, nitrogen balance in both normal and diabetic subjects was close to zero. Body weight, body composition and resting metabolic rate remained unchanged. In summary, diabetic patients are not at a higher than normal risk of malnutrition if they restrict their protein intake.

Both, type II diabetes and chronic kidney disease affect the state of insulin resistance characterized by glycemia, hyperinsulinemia, increased glucose production and decreased glucose storage and oxidation. Even if both diseases cause these metabolic disturbances in a different degree, they do have their own deleterious effects on carbohydrate metabolism. A strict protein restriction shows different positive effects on carbohydrate metabolism, known as a decrease in hepatic glucose output and gluconeogenesis as well as in post-absorptive blood glucose level and insulin concentration in normal subjects as well as in diabetic patients (IDDM and NIDDM) in a similar degree. Furthermore, the improvement of insulin sensitivity in both uremic patients and diabetic patients has been demonstrated by clamp technique.

In summary, of most importance is the kind of replacement of protein calories – as long as protein calories are made up by carbohydrate calories, reduction in protein intake improves insulin sensitivity and has beneficial influences on different steps of carbohydrate metabolism in both diabetics and normal subjects.

Dietary protein restriction has been reported to delay the need for renal replacement therapy and to reduce the rate of decline in renal function in clinical trials. Meta-analyses summarized that the effect of dietary protein restriction (0.6 g protein/kg b.w./day) was less in randomized vs. controlled trials and relatively greater among diabetic vs. non-diabetic patients. However, the number of diabetic patients studied was small and the duration of follow-up was short in most trials.

Feasibility as well as efficacy of very low protein diets supplemented with keto/amino acids have also be shown in clinical trials with diabetic and non-diabetic CKD patients. Compliance with the diet and nutritional status were not different from that found in non-diabetic uremic patients. In diabetic patients a satisfactory control of blood glucose levels with no or only minor adjustments (reduction) of insulin dosage was obtained as well as improved tissue insulin sensitivity and decreased hyperinsulinemia. These effects appear to be mediated in part by decreased production of toxic peptides acting as inhibitors of glucose utilization and decreased hepatic gluconeogenesis as well as an improvement of metabolic acidosis and secondary hyperparathyroidism. Furthermore, there is a direct effect of protein restriction on glucose metabolism as far as carbohydrates replace energy calories.

In conclusion, in diabetic patients with CKD keto/amino acid-supplemented very low protein diets have beneficial effects on the course of nephropathy without untoward effects on nutritional status. Lastly lowering of insulin resistance, reduction of hyperinsulinemia and increase in energy production rate make a keto/amino acid-supplemented very low protein diet a therapeutic arm for diabetic renal failure, particularly well adapted for the treatment of overweight or obese non-insulin-dependent diabetics with CKD.

Italy – Clinical Studies on Protein Restriction in Diabetic Nephropathy Patients – Keto Acid Therapy and Its Efficacy

Adamasco Cupisti
Pisa, Italy

Diabetic nephropathy is one of the most common causes of end stage renal disease (ESRD) in the world. According to the Italian Registry of Dialysis and Transplantation in Italy, the mean incidence of diabetic nephropathy in dialysis population is 20 pmp. Diabetic nephropathy represents the second primary renal disease in dialysis patients following vascular disease and it is still increasing within the last few years. The most important epidemiological aspect is that mortality in diabetics on renal replacement therapy (RRT) remains twofold higher than that in non-diabetics.

From this epidemiological data the need for an effective prevention of progressive nephropathy in terms of an intensive predialysis management is well evident. This includes a strict glycemic control, anti-hypertensive-antiproteinuric therapy and also nutritional treatment.

Dietary manipulation characterized by reduction of sodium, protein and phosphorus intakes and also changes in qualities of lipids and proteins are of crucial importance in the treatment of diabetic nephropathy. In this respect, the quantitative and qualitative manipulation of dietary protein is the most important feature.

It is well known that protein restriction corrects several metabolic and nutritional abnormalities and protects from progressive renal damage including prevention of glomerular hypertrophy and hyperplasia, lowering glomerular hypertension and hyperfiltration, reducing urinary protein excretion, prevention of secondary hyperparathyroidism and correction of metabolic acidosis.

According to the stage of renal disease, different dietary regimes are proposed:

1. Mild/moderate stages of chronic kidney disease (GFR >20 ml/min)

Conventional low protein diet
Protein: 0.6 g/kg b.w./day (0.4 g protein/kg b.w./day from animal origin)
Phosphorus: 8–10 mg/kg b.w./day
Energy: 30–35 kcal/kg b.w./day (7–8% protein, 30–32% lipids, 60–62% carbohydrates)
Supplements: calcium carbonate (1–2 g)

As Alternative

Vegan diet
Protein: 0.7 g/kg b.w./day from vegetable origin (cereals-legumes combination)
Phosphorus: 9–10 mg/kg b.w./day
Energy: 30–35 kcal/kg b.w./day (8% protein, 57% carbohydrates, 34% lipids: mainly complex carbohydrates, and high unsaturated/saturated fatty acid ratio)
Supplements: calcium carbonate (1–2 g), iron, vitamin B_{12}
In case of proteinuria: keto/amino acids (1 tablet/5 kg b.w./day)

2. Severe stage of chronic kidney disease (GFR <20 ml/min)

Ketodiet
Protein: 0.3–0.4 g/kg b.w./day
Phosphorus: 5–6 mg/kg b.w./day
Energy: 30–35 kcal/kg b.w./day (65% carbohydrates, 30% lipids, 4% proteins)
Supplements: keto/amino acids (1 tablet/5 kg b.w./day), calcium carbonate (1–2 g/day), vitamin B_{12}, iron.

Not only the quantity of dietary protein is of importance, but also the protein quality (i.e. from plant or animal sources). Acute and chronic renal responses to a vegetable protein and an animal protein diet are quite different. Namely, a significant increase in GRF, renal plasma flow and in fractional clearance of albumin and IgG occur during an animal protein diet, whereas no significant changes in these parameters occur following vegetable protein intake. In summary, the protein intake being equal, vegetable protein diet can reduce urinary protein excretion, prevents glomerular hyperfiltration, decreases net hydrogen production and ameliorates lipid pattern.

Available clinical results on the progression of diabetic nephropathy and metabolic and nutritional aspects indicate the efficacy of dietary protein manipulation: reduction in the mean rate of decline of creatinine clearance, significant decrease in daily urinary protein loss, good calcium-phosphate control, improvement of secondary hyperparathyroidism, a better glycemic control and reduction in the daily insulin requirements, and stability of nutritional status parameters.

It has to be emphasized that safety and efficacy of protein restriction in CKD patients is achieved by providing adequacy of essential amino acids and energy intake and correction of metabolic acidosis. In diabetic patients, strict metabolic glycemic control by an intensive treatment is necessary in order to normalize urea generation rate, net protein utilization and nitrogen balance during dietary protein restriction.

A major concern about the nutritional management is the compliance to dietary prescription. Unfortunately, the nutritional recommendations are often borrowing and offer only limited food choices. Due to this, they are not well accepted by CKD patients. Additionally the necessary number of keto/amino acid tablets is an additional obstacle for compliance. Familiar and psychological aspects should also be considered in order to achieve a good compliance. Due to this, patients should be well informed, motivated and followed-up by experienced dieticians.

In conclusion, available data regarding the Italian experience on nutritional treatment demonstrate that vegetarian low-protein regimens supplemented with essential amino/keto acids may be an useful option in the treatment of diabetic nephropathy patients as they can slow down – though not halt – the progression to ESRD, reduce urinary protein excretion, have favorable effects on calcium-phosphate metabolism and does not induce malnutrition, provided good adherence to dietary prescriptions.

Predialytic Treatment in CKD Patients

Rubén Darío Bonilla Aguirre
Guadalajara, Mexico

The main objectives in the treatment of chronic kidney disease patients are prevention of residual renal function, delay of dialytic therapy, maintenance of a suitable nutritional state and improvement of the patients' and family's life quality as well as saving institutional resources.

Up to now, the most important treatment modality of CKD patients is dialysis, associated with the highest expenses are for dialysis treatment. 60% of the monetary recourses are spending for dialysis treatment and only 10% for predialysis treatment. Nevertheless, the predialysis treatment gets an important role in the management of CKD patients.

All over the world, the most important cause of CKD is long-lasting diabetes. According to the social security (IMSS) in Mexico, 33% of CKD patients suffer from a diabetes, which means a diabetic population of 5 millions. The number of patients with diabetic nephropathy is estimated to about 625,000.

Due to the fact that patients with diabetes and/or hypertension are at a higher risk of developing chronic kidney disease, in these patients a prevention and early detection of the disease should be in the primary focus (1st level of treatment). Human resources for the integral attention of the disease include physicians, nutritionists, nurses, social workers and – of course – the patient and his familiar environment, who have to work as a well-educated health team. At the same time, material resources are required like human power, didactic resources as well as reagents and tools for diagnostic and drugs.

For patients with diabetes and/or hypertension for more than 5 years, a regular screening – starting with detection of micro- (<299 mg/24 h) or macro-albuminuria (>300 mg/24 h) should be advised. Depending on the excess of albuminuria, strategies for prevention or delaying the progression during early stages of the disease are in the focus of treatment.

According to the stage of chronic kidney disease, different treatment strategies are recommended (see table).

In Mexico, peritoneal and hemodialysis treatment are the most common treatment modalities in CKD patients, even in those with GFR about 15–20 ml/min. Unfortunately, clinical characteristics of peritoneal dialysis and hemodialysis patients are not very positive, including malnutrition, high mortality, lack of rehabilitation, frequent hospitalizations and short survival. Furthermore, these treatments absorb a huge amount of the health care

Stage of CKD	Treatment strategies
GFR 90–55 ml/min	Glucose control (<125 mg/dl) Blood pressure control (125/75 mmHg) (e.g. enalapril, verapamil, losartan) Control of metabolites (e.g. uric acid) and lipid profile Dietary protein restriction: 0.8 g/kg ideal b.w./day Exercise
GFR 54–25 ml/min	Glucose control (<125 mg/dl) Blood pressure control (125/75 mmHg) (e.g. losartan, enalapril, verapamil, amlodipin) Control of metabolites (e.g. uric acid) and lipid profile Dietary protein restriction: 0.6 g/kg ideal b.w./day and Ketosteril® EPO, calcitriol, etc. Exercise
GFR 24–10 ml/min	Glucose control (<125 mg/dl) Blood pressure control (125/75 mmHg) (e.g. losartan, enalapril, verapamil, amlodipin) Control of metabolites (e.g. uric acid) and lipid profile Dietary protein restriction: 0.4 g/kg ideal b.w./day and Ketosteril® EPO, calcitriol, etc. Exercise
GFR <10 ml/min	Glucose control (<125 mg/dl) Blood pressure control (125/75 mmHg) (e.g. losartan, enalapril, verapamil, amlodipin) Treatment of hyperlipidemia, hyperparathyroidism Dialytic treatment Dietary protein intake: 1.2–1.4 g/kg ideal b.w./day EPO, etc.

budget. Due to this, pre-dialysis management is seen as the best alternative in the management of CKD patients.

Consensus
Keto Acid Therapy for Patients with Diabetic Nephropathy

Due to the exponential growth of diabetic nephropathy (as one major cause of end-stage renal disease) alternative conventional strategies – including Keto Acid Therapy – for the treatment of diabetic nephropathy are absolutely indicated.

Keto Acid Therapy as part of a treatment program in diabetic nephropathy patients based on published literature is considered to be entirely safe and efficacious.

In diabetic nephropathy patients, a proper implementation of Keto Acid Therapy

- Does not induce malnutrition or even improve nutritional status (e.g. albumin, BMI)
- Can improve metabolic abnormalities associated with renal insufficiency (e.g. bicarbonate, phosphorus, calcium)
- Can improve/correct diabetes associated metabolic disturbances in type II (good glycemic control, improvement of insulin sensitivity, reduction of hyperinsulinemia)
- Enables a good glycemic control in type I diabetes mellitus
- May slow progression of renal insufficiency and will delay the time until dialysis is required to treat uremic symptoms

Specific international guidelines and recommendations for Keto Acid Therapy

- Low protein diet (0.6–0.7 g protein/kg b.w./day) is indicated at a creatinine clearance of 50 ml/min/1.73 m^2, Keto Acid Therapy is indicated at a creatinine clearance of 20–25 ml/min/1.73 m^2
- Daily protein intake at a low protein diet supplemented with keto acids should not exceed 0.6 g/kg b.w./day, optimal protein intake is 0.4–0.6 g/kg b.w./day
- Recommended dosage of keto acids (Ketosteril®) is 0.1 g/kg b.d./day
- Daily energy intake of 35 kcal/kg b.w./day should be recommended
- Protein calories must be replaced by complex carbohydrate calories – not by lipids

Crucial aspects for the efficacy of Keto Acid Therapy in diabetic nephropathy patients:

- Patients have to be properly selected in respect to motivation and ability to follow a protein-restricted diet
- In order to reap the benefits for diabetic nephropathy patients, it is absolutely necessary that all disciplines involved in the treatment (nephrologists/physicians/dieticians/nutritionists) act as a highly motivated team
- Support for increasing patients' compliance is needed: recipes, dietary computer program
- Development of guidelines as well as convincing Diabetes Associations/Diabetologists about the efficacy and safety of Keto Acid Therapy is regarded as a major issue for increasing the awareness of Keto Acid Therapy

Keto Acid Supplementation in Patients Being Treated by Dialysis

Nutritional Requirement during Long-Term Dialysis Treatment and Nutritional Status of Dialysis Patients – What Is the Optimal Amount of Protein?

Sergio Draibe
São Paulo, Brazil

Low nutrient intake
• Uremic anorexia
• Dialysis procedure
• Acidemia
• Intercurrent illnesses
• Gastrointestinal disorders
• Depression/oth psych dis
• Brain diseases
• Socioeconomic factors

Hypercatabolism
• Associate illnesses
• Inflammatory state
• HD procedure itself
• Acidemia
• Hormonal disorders

Losses during the procedure
• Amino acids (10–12g)
• Peptides
• Proteins (1–3g)
• Glucose (12–25g with gluc-free dialysate)

Adapted from NKF K/DOQI 2000

Fig. 1. Causes of malnutrition in hemodialysis patients.

Protein-energy malnutrition that is well recognized as an important predictor of clinical outcome in chronic dialysis patients is present in 20–50% of this population.

Actually, there is no universally accepted definition for the term 'malnutrition' in dialysis patients. Malnutrition is defined as poor nutritional status due to improper nutritional intake. However, malnutrition is generally a misdiagnosis for dialysis patients that present complex mechanism abnormalities stimulated by renal insufficiency that more commonly lead to loss of body weight and protein stores. Recently, this unique form of malnutrition related to uremia-induced complications has been suggested as 'uremic malnutrition'.

Malnutrition occurs due to pre-established deficits, acidosis, anorexia, protein/amino acid losses, and co-morbid conditions including inflammation (fig. 1).

The Outpatient Clinic of the Nephrology Division of the Federal University of São Paulo analyzed the spontaneous food intake and nutritional parameters of CKD patients divided into quartiles according to their creatinine clearance (CrCl) (<19.9 ml/min/1.73 m^2 to >43 ml/min/1.73 m^2). At the first visit, the patients' protein intake estimated by protein equivalent of nitrogen appearance was significantly lower in the first and second quartiles in comparison to the third and fourth. Energy intake was significantly lower in the first quartile when compared with the fourth. Furthermore, in patients with a CrCl of <19.9 ml/min/1.73 m^2 – characterized as a stage of CKD just before starting dialysis – signs of malnutrition were evident in a substantial proportion of patients. Thus, even before the commencement of the dialysis treatment uremic malnutrition is yet present.

Hemodialysis procedure per se has been implicated as a potential catabolic factor predisposing the chronic hemodialysis patients to protein-energy malnutrition. First of all, amino acid losses occur in the range of 8–12 g per session. Furthermore, hemodialysis can be seen as an overall catabolic event, decreasing circulating amino acids, accelerating rates of whole-body and muscle proteolysis, stimulating muscle release of amino acids, and elevating net whole body and muscle protein loss.

Elements of over-nutrition, such as increased weight, which are deleterious in the general population, paradoxically are protective in dialysis patients. Conversely, a low body mass index is a risk factor for poor outcome, i.e. high mortality in dialysis-dependent populations. These reverses or paradoxical relationships between nutritional markers and outcome have been referred as 'reverse epidemiology'.

The major question remains: what is the dietary protein requirement in maintenance hemodialysis patients in order to guarantee neutral or positive nitrogen balance? The measurement of nitrogen balance is the classic method by which dietary protein requirement is assessed. However, there are a limited number of nitrogen balance studies in hemodialysis patients.

In normal subjects, short- and long-term studies suggest that nitrogen balances are neutral with dietary protein intakes of 0.6 g/kg b.w./day. Taking account the variability of these measurements, the WHO recommends a safe level of 0.75 g/kg b.w./day.

The few metabolic studies performed in hemodialysis patients showed that neutral or positive nitrogen balances may be attained with protein intakes ranging from 0.87 to 1.13 g/kg b.w./day and a sufficient intake of calories. Concepts of an 'average' and 'safe' dietary protein intake that will maintain protein balance in almost all (97.5%) individuals are used by FAO/WHO/National Academy of Science. They have added 25% to the average protein intake to obtain safe protein intake. Taken together, the NKF-KDOQI group has recommended a dietary protein intake of about 1.2 g/kg b.w./day to ensure neutral positive nitrogen balance in stable hemodialysis patients. At least 50% of the protein ingested should be of high biological value. Energy intake of 30 to 35 kcal/kg b.w./day seems to be enough to assure neutral or positive nitrogen balance in the majority of studies.

Recommended dietary nutrient intake for adult patients undergoing maintenance hemodialysis:

Macro-/micronutrients	Recommended intake
Dietary protein intake (DPI)	1.2 g/kg b.w./day (at least 50% of the dietary protein should be of high biologic value) 1.2 to 1.3 g/kg/day for acutely ill patients
Dietary energy intake (DEI)	35 kcal/kg b.w./day: ≤60 years 30–35 kcal/kg b.w./day: ≥60 years
Total fat intake	30% of total energy intake
Saturated fat	up to 10% of total calories
Polyunsaturated fatty acids	up to 10% of total calories
Monounsaturated fatty acids	up to 20% of total calories
Carbohydrate	rest of non-protein calories
Total fiber	20–25 g/day
Sodium	750–2,000 mg/day
Potassium	up to 70–80 mEq/day
Phosphorus	10–17 mg/kg/day
Calcium	≤1,000 mg/day
Magnesium	200–300 mg/day
Iron	?
Zinc	15 mg/day
Water	usually 750–1,500 ml/day

Metabolic derangements in CKD patients associated with diabetes mellitus, secondary hyperparathyroidism and inflammation may interfere with the energy balance – examined as resting energy expenditure. It has been shown that these metabolic disturbances may increase the resting energy expenditure of the patients. Additionally to these observations, anorexia, co-morbid conditions and consequently reduction of food intake might be an explanation for the observed lower daily energy and protein intakes. Due to this, a substantial proportion of patients will need to increase their habitual protein intake. Furthermore, treatment strategies for malnourished patients in form of intravenous or oral supplementations (together with exercise) are necessary.

In conclusion, it has to be mentioned that there is controversy about the question whether dietary protein intake more than 1.2 g/kg b.w./day for hemodialysis patients is adequate. Recent studies with stable hemodialysis patients showed an increased fat mass, hyperkalemia and an accumulation of uremic toxins with graded protein intakes. Patients with a protein intake greater than 1.3 g/kg b.w./day satisfied the criterion of visceral obesity. Due to this, new treatment strategies – such as keto/amino acid supplementation during dialysis should be evaluated and discussed.

Clinical Studies on Keto/Amino Acid Supplementation of Dialysis Patients

Gabor Zakar

Székesfehérvár, Hungary

Malnutrition is a well-recognized co-morbid condition in dialysis patients that contributes to the increased mortality seen in these patients. In most cases predialysis and dialysis patients have no dietary intervention. During predialysis period, diets are characterized as uncontrolled, rather than controlled low protein diets. In dialysis patients, an increased protein intake is associated with an increased load of nitrogen and phosphate. It is recommended due to catabolic conditions and amino acid losses in the dialysate.

Malnutrition can be characterized by markers like body weight, body mass index (BMI), skinfold thicknesses and circumferences, biochemical markers (e.g. serum albumin, cholesterol, serum creatinine, urea) and subjective global assessment (SGA), known as a semiquantitative scale with three severity levels as well as modified more quantitative scoring systems (e.g. 'Hungarian Scale', malnutrition score 1995, 8-35 Kalantar-Zadeh 1999).

Multiple interventions have been tried in an effort to decrease mortality. This includes the application of protein-carbohydrate mixtures (per os/tube), intradialytic parenteral nutrition (IDPN), total parenteral nutrition, peritoneal applications and keto/amino acid preparates, which have been used as nutritional repletion in severely malnourished dialysis patients.

Oral nutritional supplementation can be used in malnourished hemodialysis patients, even if there are limited trials evaluating their efficacy. Available results indicate that oral nutritional supplements increase caloric, protein and fluid intakes, but also nitrogen and phosphorus load. These increased intakes are associated with improvement of nutritional markers in malnourished hemodialysis patients.

Intradialytic parenteral nutrition (IDPN) is a therapy that has become popular but is discussed controversial, too. Criteria for the initiation of an IDPN are serum albumin <34 g/l, unintentional loss of body weight >10%, insufficient protein (<1 g/kg b.w./day)/caloric intakes (<25 kcal/kg b.w./day), SGA 'B' or 'C' rating, PCR (<1 g/kg b.w./day) and documented gastrointestinal disorders (gastroparesis, malabsorption). Furthermore, IDPN may represent a useful form of nutritional support in the malnourished dialysis patient who has no other active disease processes, cannot ingest adequate nutrition by mouth, and has a contra-indication to or a serious complication from enteral feeding. Concerning the efficacy, results of the available literature indicate that the data supporting the use of IDPN are weak. IDPN use in hemodialysis patients seems to be associated with an improved patient outcome measured by hospitalization rate and a decrease in mortality in certain subgroups. IDPN therapy significantly increased body weight and serum albumin levels in malnourished dialysis patients. Adverse effects consisted primarily of excess fluid gain and hyperglycemia.

Peritoneal dialysis fluid containing amino acids (1.1%) has been introduced recently to improve the nutritional status of continuous ambulatory peritoneal dialysis patients. The use of amino acid dialysate has been shown to improve nutritional status (albumin levels, anthropometrics) and decrease mortality rate of malnourished peritoneal dialysis patients. The available data suggest that amino acid dialysate can be used safely and effectively for an extended period of time. Nevertheless, adverse effects like nausea and acidosis can be observed during the treatment with amino acid dialysate.

Keto/amino acid supplementation is considered as an effective alternative to the other mentioned nutritional treatment strategies. Keto/amino acid supplements represent an additional source of oral amino acids for compensation of losses, but they seem to be modulators as well. Certain keto acids are strongly interacting with nitrogen, carbohydrate and lipid metabolism. Even if there are not that many clinical studies available, keto/amino acids are well tolerated (without relevant side-effects) and improve nutritional status of dialysis patients.

In 1995, the Hungarian Nephrological Society prepared a guideline for keto/amino acid treatment of predialysis and dialysis patients. Indications for keto/amino acid treatment (1 tablet Ketosteril®/5 kg ideal b.w./day) in dialysis patients are signs of malnutrition (serum albumin <35 g/l, SGA score >8/24, if oral supplementation measures failed) on start of dialysis and/or during dialysis treatment. The Hungarian Ketosteril® Cohort Study (1995–1997) has shown that nutritional status in dialysis patients can be corrected (increase in serum albumin and an improvement in SGA scores) and PTH levels can be reduced due to a supplementation of keto/amino acids. Furthermore, first results showed that daily erythropoietin dosages in dialysis patients were reduced by the supplementation of keto/amino acids. At the moment, 435 patients in 52 Hungarian Centers use keto acids (Ketosteril®) during dialysis treatment.

In summary, future studies are needed in order to evaluate comparative outcome data on mortality and cardiovascular morbidity as well as comparative data with other types of nutritional support.

Consensus

Keto Acid Supplementation in Patients Being Treated by Dialysis

It is estimated that 30–50% of dialysis patients suffer from protein-energy malnutrition. Nutritional status is an important predictor of clinical outcome in chronic hemodialysis patients, as uremic malnutrition is strongly associated with an increased risk of death and hospitalization events. Abnormalities in nutritional markers are common and include decreased serum protein/albumin, lower body mass as assessed by anthropometric measurements and subjective global assessment, and decreased nutrient intake. In this context, a decreased muscle mass is the most significant predictor of morbidity and mortality in these patients.

Oral supplementation of keto/amino acids in dialysis patients may have beneficial effects in

- Compensation of essential amino acids being lost into the dialysate
- Normalization of low plasma levels of amino acids, especially branched-chain amino acids
- Improvement overall nutritional status (albumin, SGA, body weight) in malnourished dialysis patients
- Supporting the normalization of calcium-phosphate disorders (increasing serum calcium and reducing phosphate levels)

Recommendations for protein and energy intake and keto/amino acid supplementation in patients being treated by dialysis:

- Dietary protein intake: 1.2 g/kg b.w./day
- Dietary energy intake: 35 kcal/kg b.w./day: ≤60 years 30–35 kcal/kg b.w./day: ≥60 years
- Recommended dosage of keto acids (Ketosteril®): 1 tablet/5–8 kg b.w./day

Central needs in order to judge the efficacy of keto/amino acid supplementation in patients being treated by dialysis are studies. In case keto/amino acids could induce lean body mass (e.g. measured by DEXA or other equivalent measures), it would be a real alternative for nutritional repletion in malnourished patients.